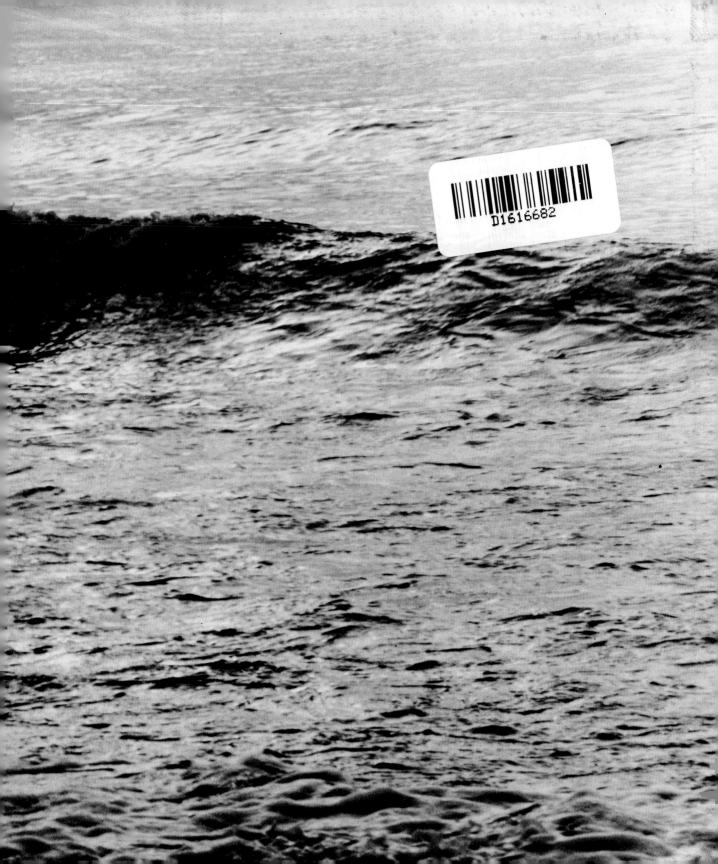

Atlas of Aquatic Dermatology

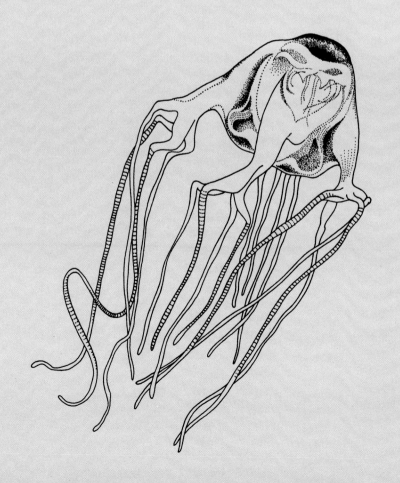

Atlas of
Aquatic
Dermatology

Alexander A. Fisher, M.D.

Clinical Professor, Department of Dermatology
New York University Post-Graduate Medical School

Associate Attending in Dermatology
University Hospital
New York University Medical Center
New York, New York

GRUNE & STRATTON
A Subsidiary of Harcourt Brace Jovanovich, Publishers
New York   San Francisco   London

This special edition is distributed by
LEDERLE LABORATORIES
as a service to the Continuing
Education of Medical Specialists
in Dermatology and Allergy.

Grune & Stratton, Inc.
111 Fifth Avenue
New York, New York 10003

Distributed in the United Kingdom by
Academic Press, Inc. (London) Ltd.
24/28 Oval Road, London NW 1

Library of Congress Catalog Card Number 78−67182
International Standard Book Number 0-8089-1139-2

Printed in the United States of America

The inclusion in text of product-related information does not
imply endorsement by the author of products of Lederle
Laboratories, nor is there any intent to suggest or imply their
use for any condition discussed unless it is specifically
mentioned in the labelling.

Produced by Creative Annex, Inc.

I wish to thank all my colleagues who so generously contributed photographic materials. Particular thanks to W. L. Orris, formerly Director of Medical Services, Scripps Institution of Oceanography, for his cooperation and assistance.

A.A.F.

Contents

Maps and Illustrations

Introduction

It is paradoxical that, in our age of modern technological advance and myriad amusements, man's primitive urge for sea and surf actually seems to be accelerating.

According to estimates, approximately 80 per cent of the world's population will have migrated to coastal areas by the year 2000. Many Americans are drawn to the water—both coastal and inland—for recreational purposes.

A 1975 report from the National Oceanic and Atmospheric Administration indicates that there are some three million recreational divers and one million commercial, military and scientific divers in the United States today. Add to this the untold numbers of swimmers, surfers, snorklers, water skiers, and fishing and boating enthusiasts, and one can begin to appreciate the lure that our fresh and salt waters hold for millions of Americans.

Little wonder, then, that water-related injuries and diseases have shown a precipitate increase from year to year and that aquatic medicine has developed as a specialty in its own right. Much recent attention has been given to "scuba sickness" (air embolism, decompression sickness) and its attendant hyperbaric therapies. On the other hand, the important field of aquatic dermatology has been comparatively neglected—despite the empiric observations of both coastal and inland dermatologists throughout the country that they are seeing more and more patients with water-related dermatoses.

Our oceans, lakes, swamps, swimming pools—and even fish tanks—contain numerous creatures and plants, large and small, as well as a multitude of microscopic organisms. Many of these water organisms have evolved self-protective stinging, biting and envenomating mechanisms capable of producing unique and various skin eruptions, along with occasional systemic reactions.

In addition to the considerable variety of water-related skin manifestations, management of aquatic dermatoses is further complicated by the much-discussed mobility of modern man. Patients jet to distant locales on vacation or business, immerse themselves in strange oceans, lakes and rivers—and frequently return with "imported" water-related skin lesions. Since some of the skin manifestations do not appear for weeks or even months, the dermatologist in Connecticut or Kansas may well be required to manage an unfamiliar condition originating in Bermuda or Aruba. By the same token, the patient presenting to a California or Idaho dermatologist with an apparent water-related dermatosis may have recently returned from the Great Lakes region—a frequent source of cercarial dermatitis produced by freshwater schistosomes.

Although many of these conditions are self-limiting, they nevertheless require attention. Appropriate first aid treatment is certainly indicated for such symptoms as pruritus, painful lesions, bullae or wounds. More important, related systemic pathology can lead to disastrous consequences if left untreated. A high index of suspicion is essential. In many instances, prompt and accurate diagnosis is vital and even life-saving.

Until publication of this volume, dermatologists have had to cope with water-related dermatoses without benefit of a basic reference work. Outside of a brief chapter in my book on *Contact Dermatitis* (Lea and Febiger, 1973), extensively organized material on the subject is virtually nonexistent in the medical literature. Exposure to this growing field of aquatic dermatology is also quite sparse in medical school or during residency.

Clearly the time is ripe for a single, central reference work dealing with water-related dermatoses, and this *Atlas of Aquatic Dermatology* has been prepared to fulfill this need.

Here the practicing dermatologist will find discussions of such diverse dermatoses as *swimmers' itch, sea bathers' eruption, creeping eruption, trench foot, aquagenic urticaria* and *swimming and fish tank granulomas.* The effects of venoms, stings, bites and spines of various aquatic organisms are thoroughly elucidated.

This *Atlas* is meant to serve a three-fold purpose: 1) to acquaint the physician with the etiologic factors of aquatic dermatitis; 2) to portray in word and photograph the clinical appearance of various aquatic dermatoses as an aid to differential diagnosis; and 3) to provide the physician with pertinent therapeutic information, enabling him to institute the most current means of managing the manifold forms of aquatic dermatitis.

Photographs of both water organisms and clinical symptoms are provided. In addition, the usefulness of this *Atlas of Aquatic*

Dermatology has been enhanced by the inclusion of a geographic cross-index of dermatosis-producing aquatic organisms. By utilizing the text and photographs as well as the geographic index, the clinician can not only feel confident in managing the protean forms of aquatic dermatitis and injury, but also have a specific basis on which to advise patients who plan to enter unfamiliar waters.

Dermatitis Caused by the Portuguese Man-of-War, Jellyfish, and Related Coelenterates

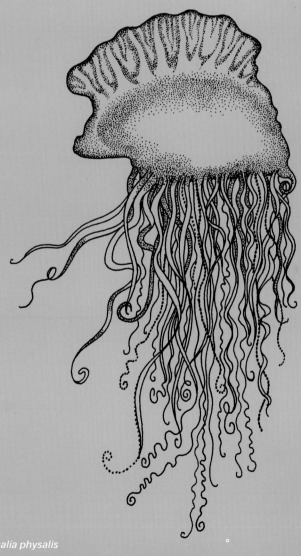

Portuguese man-of-war *Physalia physalis*

Dermatitis Caused by the Portuguese Man-of-War, Jellyfish, and Related Coelenterates

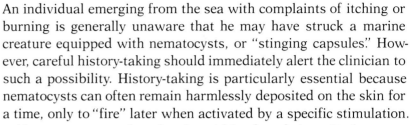

An individual emerging from the sea with complaints of itching or burning is generally unaware that he may have struck a marine creature equipped with nematocysts, or "stinging capsules." However, careful history-taking should immediately alert the clinician to such a possibility. History-taking is particularly essential because nematocysts can often remain harmlessly deposited on the skin for a time, only to "fire" later when activated by a specific stimulation.

Nematocysts are found only within the phylum Coelenterata. Coelenterates are radially symmetrical animals of simple structure. The mouth opens into a single cavity, and the body wall is formed by two layers of cells with structureless jelly between them. Almost all coelenterates possess nematocysts. These "stinging capsules" are especially concentrated on the tentacles.

This large and variegated phylum is particularly abundant in all tropical and subtropical waters. Of the 9,000 or so species that have been identified, approximately 100—including jellyfishes, sea anemones, fire corals, and the Portuguese man-of-war—are capable of producing injuries to man. The classes within this phylum and several clinically significant species are shown in Table 1-1.

Most dreaded of the coelenterates is the Portuguese man-of-war, a creature whose ominous character has assumed almost legendary proportions. While the effects of contact with the Portuguese man-of-war (discussed later) may be severe, its sting is rarely fatal. In fact, the most dangerous of the coelenterates appear to be several of the Australian Cubomedusae: the carybdeid "irukandju," and the chiropropids *Chironex fleckeri* and *Chiropsalmus quadrigatus*.[1]

The Nature of Nematocysts

These dead organoids—also known as "nettle cells" in addition to "stinging capsules"—contain the toxic substance of the coelenterate.

Each nematocyst contains a spirally-coiled thread with a barbed end. Upon contact, this thread is uncoiled and forcibly ejected—along with a toxin—into the skin. The size of the barb and the toxic substance it introduces vary widely in different species.

The stimulation necessary to discharge a nematocyst apparently involves both chemical and mechanical factors. It has been shown that freshwater stimulates the "firing" of nematocysts. Friction may also cause nematocysts to "fire," and patients suspected of

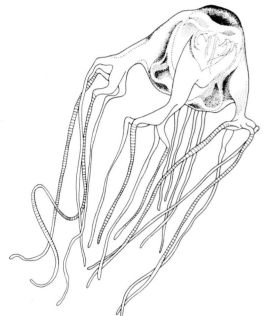

To prevent dormant nematocysts (stinging capsules, nettle cells) remaining on the skin from "firing," patients should:

1. Avoid contact with freshwater.

2. Avoid rubbing affected area.

Fig. 1-1.

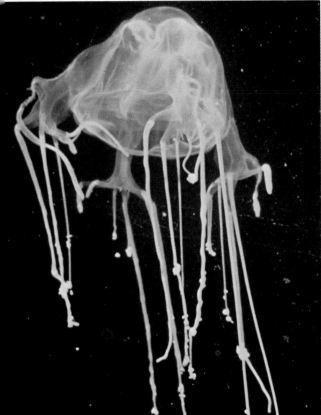

Fig. 1-1. *CHIRONEX FLECKERI,* found primarily off the northern coast of Australia, is also seen in the Caribbean, the Gulf of Mexico and off the Atlantic coasts of North and South America. Fatalities are said to ensue in 15 to 20% of stingings. Courtesy of Bruce W. Halstead, M.D.

Fig. 1-2. *SEA ANEMONE.* All species in this group of phylum Coelenterata, class Anthozoa, have nematocysts. Because of their variety of colors, animal sea anemones frequently have a flower-like appearance similar to plant anemones. They are not as harmless, however, as their botanical name-sakes because they can cause dermatitis. Other sea anemones produce dermatitis by a sting rather than by nematocysts. Courtesy of Michael D. Rosco, M.D.

Fig. 1-3. *PHYSALIA PHYSALIS* drags numerous fishing tentacles containing bead-like batteries of nematocysts along their entire length. Since the tentacles of this hydroid sometimes reach a length of 100 feet, swimmers can be severely stung even at a distance from the animal. The stinging capsules penetrate the skin and inject a fluid containing a neurotoxin. Courtesy of Bruce W. Halstead, M.D.

Fig. 1-3.

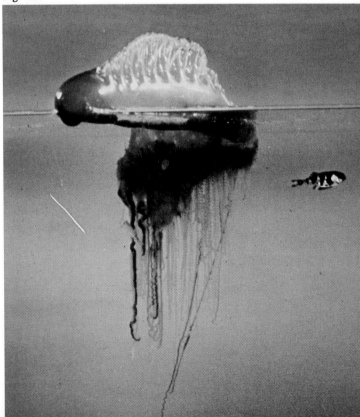

Fig. 1-2.

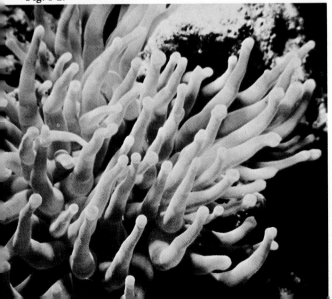

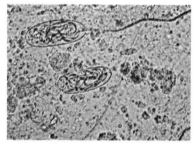

Fig. 1-4. *NEMATOCYSTS* of the
phylum Coelenterata are dead organoids. Also known as "nettle cells" or
"stinging capsules," they contain the
toxic substance.
Courtesty of Bruce W. Halstead, M.D.

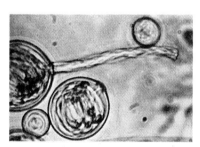

Fig. 1-5. *PHYSALIA NEMATOCYSTS.*
Each nematocyst contains a spirally-
coiled thread with a barbed end. Upon
contact this thread is uncoiled (as
seen here) and forcibly ejected along
with a toxin into the skin.
Courtesy of H. L. Arnold, Jr., M.D.

being contaminated with nematocysts should be advised to avoid
rubbing or scratching affected areas.

Nematocyst Venom

High molecular weight toxins isolated from coelenterates have been
shown to be heat labile, nondialyzable, and degraded by proteolytic
agents. In many animal species, these toxins appear to inhibit
nerve activity by altering ionic permeability. The toxins may also
induce cardiac dysfunction.

Experimental studies have shown that animals contacting or
receiving the venom parenterally experience severe pain and paralysis in the central nervous system soon after envenomization. Other
sequelae may include urticaria, pruritus, edema, paralysis, cardiac
arrest, and death.

A toxic protein-tetramine complex seems to be operative in coelenterate extracts. Paralysis and central nervous system effects
appear to be primarily related to toxic proteins and peptides and
secondarily to the presence of tetramine. Burning pain and urticaria
can probably be explained by the presence of serotonin, histamine,
or histamine-releasing agents in the venom.

Range of Dermatologic Reactions*

Dermatitis resulting from contact with nematocyst-containing tentacles varies with the concentration of stings and the toxicity of the
venom. The severity ranges from a mild stinging to a marked burning sensation. There is usually a linear, papular eruption accompanied by erythema and edema. Severe dermatitis may be accompanied by pain and marked itching.[2]

Urticarial eruptions possibly accompanied by anaphylactic
reactions—pronounced weakness, edema of the throat and larynx
—occur with some frequency. Shock and death may ensue in children and in those with exceptional hypersensitivity.

Principles of Treatment†

In the past, various recommendations for the alleviation of coelenterate stings included the application of vinegar, alcohol, ammonia,
urine, ice water, hot water, potassium permanganate crystals, formalin, barnacle juice and meat tenderizer.

Current responsible opinion would seem to indicate the following measures:

1. Avoid the use of freshwater, as it activates nematocysts. Never allow the victim to enter a fresh shower after exposure to a coelenterate until the nematocyst toxin has been neutralized. The result could be extreme intensification of symptoms, even shock. The patient's skin may, however, be gently rinsed with *seawater* without adverse effect.

2. Apply alcohol to inactivate the toxin introduced by the nematocyst. Virtually any type of alcohol available is adequate, including rubbing alcohol, liquor, toilet water, cologne, or perfume. Make sure the alcohol is applied over the affected areas.

3. Alternatively, apply proteolytic meat tenderizers. These act in a similar fashion to alcohol.

4. Avoid formalin, which is too toxic for routine use.

5. If nothing else is available, salt water heated to the limit of tolerance may help neutralize the venom.

6. To help remove clinging tentacles, a paste of seawater and baking soda may be applied five minutes after the alcohol. Application of flour or talcum will serve the same purpose, coalescing the tentacles, which may then be readily scraped off with a knife or sharp instrument. Dry sand may be used if powders are not available. (Tentacles should not be removed with the ungloved hand.)

7. Wash the areas again with salt water.

8. In severe cases—especially if the victim is a child—tourniquets on the exposed limbs may be lifesaving. The purpose of the tourniquet is *not* to stop arterial flow, but to reduce venous return. Always use a rubber tourniquet and apply it so that a finger can

First aid treatment of coelenterate stings:
1. Detoxify with alcohol or meat tenderizer (papain).
2. Coalesce tentacles with talcum powder and scrape off.
3. Treat shock with epinephrine and corticosteroids.

*Reactions caused by specific coelenterates are detailed later in this chapter.

†In addition to these general treatment procedures, specific therapeutic measures may be necessary to counteract the nematocysts of certain coelenterates. These are described in the appropriate subsection. Wherever discussion of specific measures is absent, the reader can assume that the general treatment regimen is appropriate.

Fig. 1-6. *CHRONEX FLECKERI STING.* Severe dermatitis in a four-year-old boy stung by the sea wasp. The sting of this sea wasp ultimately proved fatal. Courtesy of J.H. Barnes, M.D.

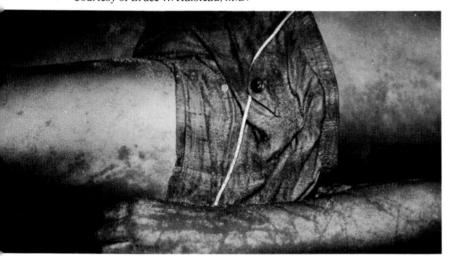

Fig. 1-7. *CHIRONEX FLECKERI STING.* Another sea wasp fatality in a ten-year-old boy. *Chironex fleckeri* causes more fatalities than any other member of the phylum Coelenterata. Even in non-fatal cases, a severe dermatitis may result. Courtesy of Bruce W. Halstead, M.D.

Fig. 1-9. *PORTUGUESE MAN-OF-WAR STING.* After contact with the tentacles, the patient experienced a severe stinging sensation, accompanied by burning numbness and severe paresthesia. Characteristically, the skin inflammation in these cases is demonstrated by linear urticarial lesions, which occasionally ulcerate. After the erythema and edema subside, vesicular dermatitis often follows. The vesicular eruption may resemble poison ivy dermatitis, particularly when the eruption is linear. Courtesy of Douglas Marsland, M.D.

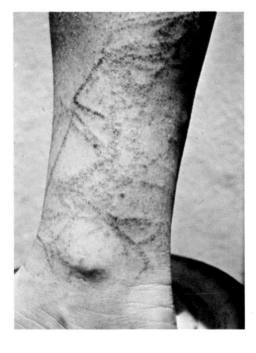

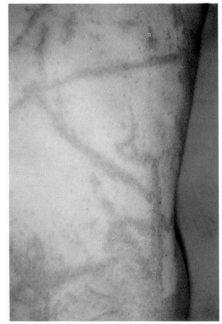

Fig. 1-8. *CHIROPSALMUS QUADRIGATUS DERMATITIS* of the leg. A severe linear vesicular eruption, the linear lesions are sites where the tentacles came in contact with the leg. Courtesy of J. H. Barnes, M.D.

be slipped underneath. Release the tourniquet for three or four minutes every hour.

9. Treat shock with epinephrine and systemic corticosteroids.

10. Use local anesthetic ointments, creams, lotions or aerosols to alleviate burning or pruritus. (Avoid benzocaine preparations. Instead employ lidocaine derivatives.)

11. Clean ulcerating lesions three times a day. Apply an antiseptic ointment, preferably one containing erythromycin or tetracycline, which are generally not sensitizing.

12. Secondary infections are relatively rare. The use of antibiotics is usually limited to patients in whom a large cutaneous area is involved. (I find that most secondary infections caused by marine ulcerations usually respond to erythromycin or tetracycline.)

13. Treat acute pain with a combination of aspirin, phenacetin, and codeine.

Portuguese Man-of-War Dermatitis

The species *Physalia physalis,* the Portuguese man-of-war, is perhaps the best known of the free-floating coelenterates. This large and rather awesome creature inhabits subtropical, tropical, and temperate zone waters throughout the Atlantic and as far east as the Mediterranean Sea. Related species are also found in the Pacific and Indian Oceans. Large colonies of hydroids drift on the water surface, supported by a purple bladder-like part of the colony which catches the wind and functions as a sail.

Physalia physalis drags numerous fishing tentacles containing bead-like batteries of nematocysts along their entire length. Since these tentacles sometimes reach a length of some 100 feet, swimmers can be severely stung even at a distance from the animal.[3] Upon discharge, the stinging capsules penetrate the skin and inject a fluid containing a neurotoxin. This toxin is believed to be a multicomponent system apparently made up of phospholipases A and B, several neutral lipids, enzymes with high proteolytic activity, and biologically active peptides.

After contact with the tentacles of the Portuguese man-of-war,

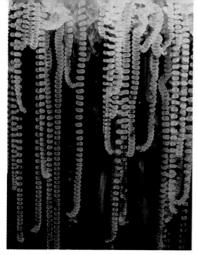

Fig. 1-10. *TENTACLES* of a Portuguese man-of-war along which the nematocysts are arranged in rows.

Detached jellyfish tentacles and those broken off during a storm may remain toxic for weeks or even months.

the patient may experience a sharp stinging sensation, burning numbness, and severe paresthesia. Skin inflammation may vary from linear urticarial lesions to ulceration. A vesicular dermatitis is a fairly common sequela following erythema, edema, itching, and burning. Children who grasp the tentacles of the Portuguese man-of-war, then cry and rub their eyes, may develop acute conjunctivitis.

Systemic manifestations—often occurring soon after contact—include lacrimation, coryza, muscular pains, dyspnea, and a feeling of constriction in the chest.

Despite the intense pain and discomfort experienced by the patient, collapse and death are relatively rare. Death may occur if the areas stung are extensive in relation to the size of the patient. Collapse is generally presaged by nausea and backache experienced 10 or 15 minutes after initial dermatologic symptoms become apparent. More commonly, recovery occurs within several hours, although the skin lesions may pass through a stage of hemorrhagic necrosis before healing. Healed lesions may leave pigmented striae for weeks or months. Permanent scarring occasionally results.[4]

Nematocysts detached from the tentacles of the Portuguese man-of-war remain capable of firing for at least several months afterward—a factor that the clinician should bear in mind when managing a patient who has come in contact with *Physalia physalis.*

"Bluebottle" Stings

Physalia utriculus, the Pacific species of the Portuguese man-of-war (known as "Bluebottle" in Australia and New Zealand) is considerably smaller than its Atlantic cousin. According to Arnold,[5] the Hawaiian species of Bluebottle rarely grows as long as three or four inches, with tentacles rarely exceeding 10 or 15 feet.

Bluebottle stings elicit dermatologic reactions similar to those of *Physalia physalis,* although symptomatology is generally less severe. Fatalities are extremely rare, and serious reactions are uncommon.

Treatment of skin lesions caused by Bluebottle stings is similar to that employed for *Physalia physalis* eruptions. Immediate lay remedies, such as rubbing with beach sand or dilute ammonia, provide some physical and psychological relief.[5]

Marr[6] reports that undischarged nematocysts and toxin can be

Table 1-1
The Phylum Coelenterata*

1. Class: **Hydrozoa**

       A. Order: Siphonophora

       Species: *Physalia physalis* (Portuguese man-of-war)
                     Velella velella

       B. Order: Calycophora (glassy nectophore)

       C. Order: Leptomedusae (feather hydroids)

       D. Order: Milleporina

       Species: *Millepora alcincornis* (stinging corals [not a
                     true coral])

2. Class: **Scyphozoa** (true jellyfish)

       A. Order: Cubomedusae (box jellies or sea wasps)

       Species: *Chironex fleckeri* (sea wasp)
                     Chiropsalmus quadrigatus

3. Class: **Anthozoa**

  Subclass: Zoantharia

       A. Order: Actiniaria (sea anemones)

       B. Order: Scleractinia (corals)

*Fisher AA: Aquatic contact dermatitis, in Fisher AA: *Contact Dermatitis*, ed 2. Philadelphia, Lea & Febiger, 1973, p 337.

inactivated by applying gasoline, ether, or alcohol, or by lathering and shaving the area of the sting.

Jellyfish Dermatitis

(Sea Nettle Dermatitis)

Jellyfish, native to both salt and freshwater, are among the most ubiquitous of sea creatures. Certain species, such as *Chironex fleckeri* ("sea wasp"), and *Cyanea* and *Chrysaora* ("sea nettles"), are extremely troublesome to man and even deadly. They are often found congregated, brought close to land or washed ashore by storms.

The small freshwater jellyfish (Craspedacusta) is similar in structure to its frequently larger salt water relatives. The main body of the salt water type is attached to trailing tentacles. These tentacles can attain considerable length in proportion to the body and are beaded with batteries of nematocysts. Even when the tentacles break away during storms, they retain their stinging toxic capabilities for two or three months.

Symptomatology varies according to the venom of a particular species, as well as to the number of nematocysts which have penetrated the victim's skin. Shock and even death may ensue if the victim is young, particularly sensitive, or stung by the deadly "sea wasp."

It is often possible to identify the species of offending jellyfish by microscopic study of the nematocysts on the patient's skin. In certain cases, identification may also be made by noting the type of eruption and the linear patterns of the lesions, one pattern being specific for a particular species of jellyfish. The initial lesions caused by *Chironex fleckeri,* for example, are multiple linear wheals with transverse bars. The purple or brown marks from the tentacles form a whiplash skin lesion.[7]

Tentacles that have become attached to the patient's skin should be removed while wearing gloves. Rinsing with seawater may also aid in the removal of tentacles and nematocysts.

A Sea Wasp Antivenin which counteracts the *Chironex fleckeri* venom is available from the Commonwealth Serum Laboratories Parkville, Victoria, Australia.

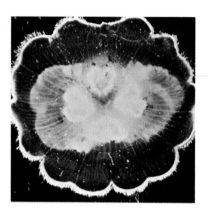

Fig. 1-11. *CASSIOPEDAL JELLYFISH* produces mild stings. It is found most often in Florida and the West Indies. Courtesy of Bruce W. Halstead, M.D.

Sea Anemone Dermatitis

(Sponge Fisherman's Disease or Sponge Diver's Disease)

Animal sea anemones belong to the phylum Coelenterata, class Anthozoa. All species have nematocysts. Because of their variety of colors, animal sea anemones frequently have a flower-like appearance similar to plant anemones. Unfortunately, they are not as harmless as their botanical namesakes.

The characteristic contact dermatitis produced by a sea anemone is related to the specific toxicity of the venom of the offending species. *Actinia* induces painful urticarial reactions, whereas *Anemonia* causes an itching-burning sensation at the sting site, accompanied by swelling and erythema.[8]

The most common skin condition caused by animal sea anemones is *Sagartia* dermatitis —"Sponge Fisherman's Disease" or "la maladie des pêcheurs d'éponges nus," as it is termed in some Mediterranean areas. *Sagartia* has the shape of a flower. It is approximately 4 cm long and has a hollow polypoid cylinder with two rows of graceful tentacles radially arranged.

This small sea anemone attaches itself symbiotically to the base of sponges. When diving for sponges, nude fishermen locate them by feeling along the ocean floor with their hands. After uprooting the sponges and cleaning them by removing stones and other encrusted debris, the fisherman places the sponges in a net suspended from his neck. During such activity, sponge fishermen have ample opportunity to come in contact with the stinging tentacles of *Sagartia*.

Within a few minutes after contact, the patient experiences an itching-burning sensation, accompanied by erythema and vesicles. The lesion is initially swollen and red, changing later to a deep purple. Headache, nausea, vomiting, fever, chills, and muscle spasms are frequent complaints.

Immediate treatment is similar to that instituted for jellyfish stings, i.e., remove tentacles while wearing gloves and rinse affected area with seawater. The healing process may be relatively slow. In addition, multiple abscesses with sloughing ulcers may develop, necessitating antibiotic treatment.

Sponge Fisherman's Disease is a dermatitis produced by a coelenterate attached symbiotically to sponges.

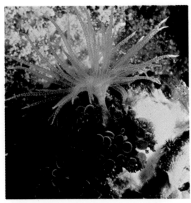

Fig. 1-12. *TRIACTIS PRODUCTA* is a venomous sea anemone endemic to the Red Sea. It is pale brown with blue fluorescence surrounding the bubble-like vesicles. The species appears to have three different types of tentacles — hence the name Triactis. However, the only true tentacles encircle the mouth. The other structures having a tentacle-like appearance are actually the hemispheric vesicles and stalked branch outgrowths.
Courtesy of David Masry, M.D. and Bruce W. Halstead, M.D.

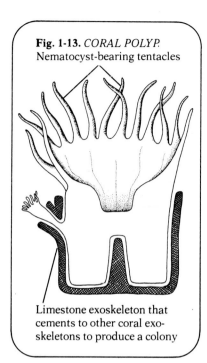

Fig. 1-13. *CORAL POLYP.*
Nematocyst-bearing tentacles

Limestone exoskeleton that cements to other coral exoskeletons to produce a colony

Coral cuts should be vigorously cleansed to remove calcareous coral particles and the wound sprinkled with antibiotic powder.

Coral Dermatitis and Coral Cuts

The skin lesions produced by the Coelenterate corals, *Milleporina*, are caused by a combination of factors—effects of the nematocyst venom, laceration by the razor-sharp exoskeleton of the coral, foreign body reaction, and secondary infection.[7] True corals are structures of various sizes and shapes, formed by the cementing of tiny limestone exoskeletons or polyps, of the order of Scleractinia.

Nematocysts of true coral are usually fairly innocuous and the resulting dermatitis—a pruritic erythema—can be effectively treated with a simple cooling lotion such as calamine lotion or alcohol.

Coral cuts should be treated vigorously to prevent secondary infection and ulceration. The following procedures are suggested:

1. Using soap and water, scrub the lesions with a soft brush or rough towel. Such vigorous cleansing is necessary to remove any calcareous pieces of coral which may become embedded in the lesion and produce an indolent wound.

2. Apply hydrogen peroxide and allow to "boil" for several minutes. Dry the wound.

3. Apply isopropyl alcohol, and sprinkle the powder contents of a capsule of tetracycline over the wound while still wet. Pat into a paste with an applicator and allow the paste to dry.

   The crust that is formed serves as a covering on the wound, remaining intact after bathing and allowing the lesion to heal from its outer edges. No bandage is necessary.

4. If the wound does not heal promptly, surgical debridement under a local anesthetic may become necessary.

Stinging or Fire Coral Dermatitis

The species *Millepora alcincornis* is not a coral at all. However, it looks like coral and acts like coral at least in one respect—it has nematocysts which cause skin eruptions. The nematocysts are located in the organism's wet mucus.

"Fire coral" is found living among true coral in the tropical Pacific Ocean, Indian Ocean, Red Sea, and Caribbean Sea. It can be recognized by its yellowish-brown color, somewhat like mustard.

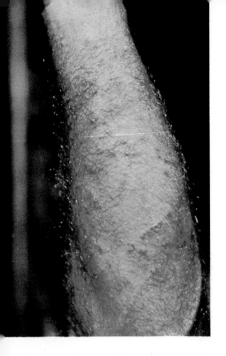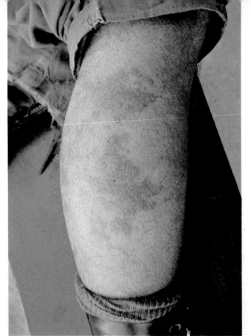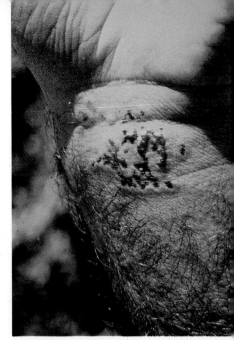

Fig. 1-14. *SEA ANEMONE STING.* Dermatitis produced by Sagartia is characterized by an initial red edematous eruption which eventually becomes deep purple. Sagartia dermatitis is the most common skin condition caused by animal sea anemones.
Courtesy of Bruce W. Halstead, M.D. and William Orris, M.D.

Fig. 1-15. *ACTINODENDRON STING.* The sting produced by this anemone, found in the tropical waters of the Pacific and Australia, is usually more localized than jellyfish stings. The resultant dermatitis is often mild, but in rare instances the reaction can be severe.
Courtesy of Bruce W. Halstead, M.D.

Fig. 1-16. *TRIACTIS PRODUCTA DERMATITIS.* The volar surface of the left wrist of a male shows the lesions produced by this sea anemone. Shortly after being stung, the local discomfort was accompanied by headache, a feeling of generalized weakness, and syncope. Moderate to severe pain continued for about five days, after which the dermatitis gradually disappeared.
Courtesy of David Masry, M.D. and Bruce W. Halstead, M.D.

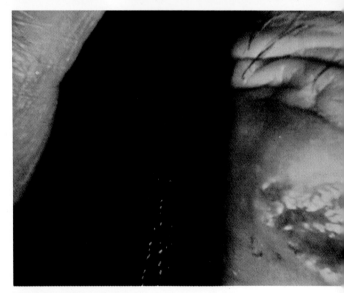

Fig. 1-17. *CORAL CUT ULCER.* Ulceration of the finger produced by a coral cut was quite deep, with rather sharp elevated borders. Granulation tissue is present in the depth of the ulcer. The ulcers are probably caused by a combination of factors, *i.e.,* a laceration by the razor sharp exoskeleton of the coral, the effects of the nemato-cyst venom, a foreign body reaction and secondary infection.
Courtesy of William Orris, M.D.

The eruption resulting from contact with stinging coral is erythematous, papular, and patchy. It appears one to ten hours after contact, usually subsiding within one to three days. Pustules may develop in severe cases.

Feather Hydroid Dermatitis

Contact dermatitis may be induced by four species of the order Leptomedusae. These "feather hydroids" are fairly abundant in tropical and subtropical waters. Swimmers climbing onto offshore rafts or swimming around pilings are most commonly afflicted by this hydrozoan.

The feather hydroid venom affects the skin more slowly than does jellyfish venom. The venom may cause two types of skin eruption: (1) urticaria developing within a few minutes after contact, or (2) delayed papular, hemorrhagic, or zosteriform reaction occurring 4 to 12 hours after contact.

Characteristic bands of dermatitis 20 cm wide may be produced, accompanied by erythema multiforme and morbilliform eruptions. The patient may experience marked anxiety and apprehension. Systemic reactions may include severe abdominal pain and muscle spasms, diarrhea, and fever. Epinephrine and systemic corticosteroids may be administered. Recovery can usually be achieved within several days.

The patient should be warned against repeated exposure to feather hydroids. Such exposure may lead to allergic sensitization, possibly resulting in anaphylactic shock.

Velella Velella Dermatitis

(By-the-Wind Sailor or Purple Sail Dermatitis)

This species of the order Siphonophora is found in the same areas as the Portuguese man-of-war. Drifting on the water much in the style of the Portuguese man-of-war, it resembles a purple-edged, thin triangular sail on an oval float. Nematocysts are contained in the trailing tentacles it uses to capture prey.

The characteristic dermatitis produced by *Velella velella* is a mild papulourticarial eruption.

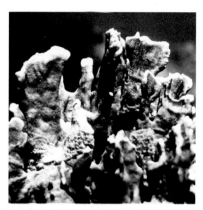

Fig. 1-18. *FIRE CORAL* or *STINGING CORAL.* While it looks like coral, *Millepora alcincornis* is not a true coral. However, it acts like coral since it has nematocysts which cause skin eruptions. These nematocysts are located in the organism's wet mucus. Courtesy of the Miami Seaquarium

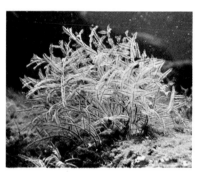

Fig. 1-19. *STINGING HYDROID.* The venom of this hydrozoan—one of four species of the order Leptomedusae that may produce dermatitis —reacts on the skin more gradually than does jellyfish venom. Courtesy of Bruce W. Halstead, M.D.

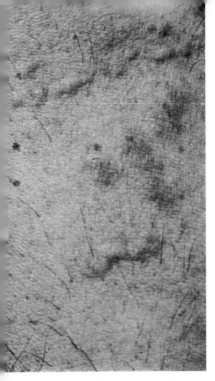

Fig. 1-20. *CARYBDEA YASTONI STING.*
A close up view of the typical linear
urticarial eruption.
Courtesy of William Orris, M.D.

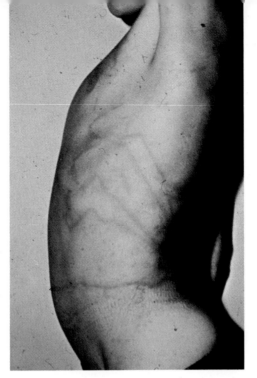

Fig. 1-21. *CYANEA CAPILLATA STING.*
The stinging hairs of a sea nettle
caused this characteristic skin pattern.
Courtesy of William Orris, M.D.

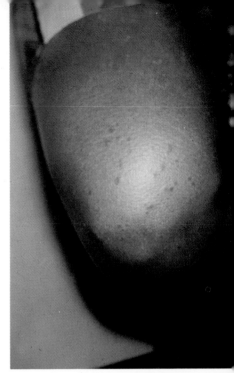

Fig. 1-22. *HYDROID DERMATITIS.*
The immediate papular urticarial type of
eruption is shown here. Occasionally,
the eruption is hemorrhagic or zosteriform, usually occurring from 4 to 12
hours after contact.
Courtesy of H.L. Arnold, M.D.

Calycophora Dermatitis
(Stinging Water Dermatitis)

Calycophora, also an order of the phylum Coelenterata, is extremely
elusive. Since the creature has almost the same index of refraction
as seawater, it can be seen only when sunlight strikes it directly.

Contact with this small, "glassy nectophore," as it is called, may
result in a markedly pruritic eruption which may persist from several hours to several days. Glassy nectophore is found particularly
in deep seawater.

"Indirect" Coelenterate Dermatitis

Before concluding this chapter, it should be noted that it may be
possible to develop coelenterate-related dermatitis without actual
direct contact with any species in the phylum. This can occur in
two ways:

Map 1-1.
Distribution of Reported Coelenterate Stings

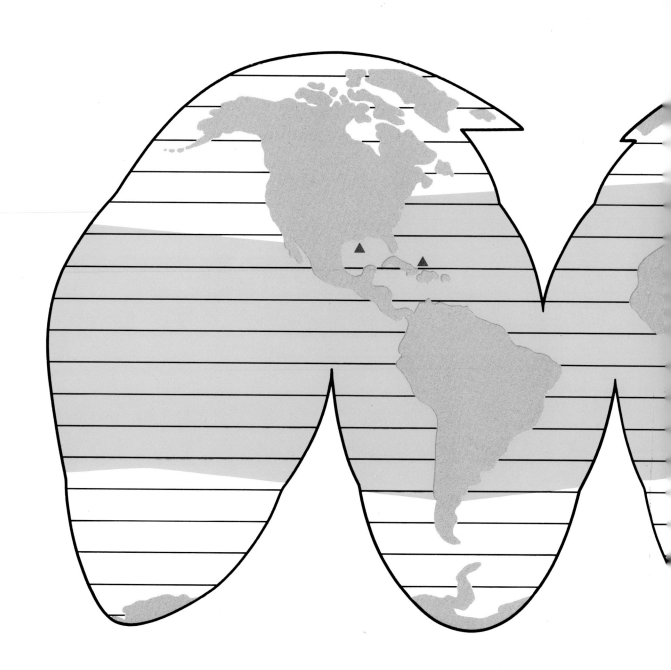

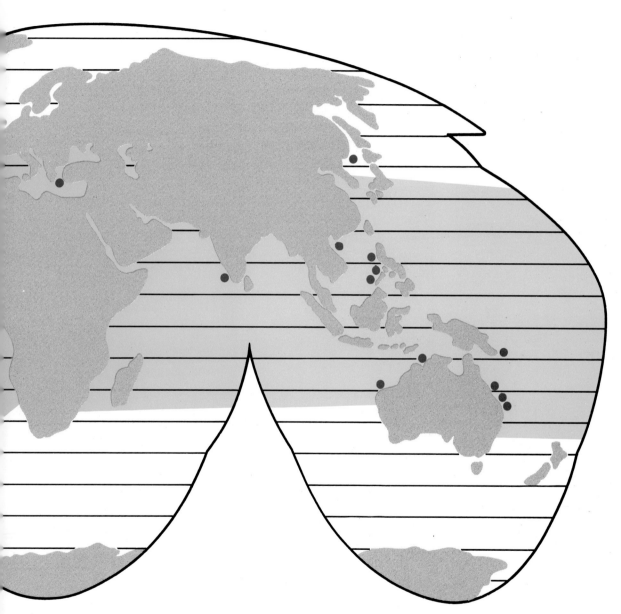

Area of greatest incidence of stings

● Fatalities due to jellyfish stings

▲ Fatalities due to Physalia stings

(Adapted from Halstead BW: Poisonous and Venomous
Marine Animals of the World. Vol 1. Washington, DC,
US Government Printing Office, 1965, p 534.)

1. Two species of nudibranch, *Glaucus atlanticus* and *Glaucus glaucilla*, eat the nematocysts and tentacles of the Portuguese man-of-war. The nematocysts pass through these sea slugs undigested and are deposited in the dorsal papillae. Bathers coming into contact with these "armed" nudibranchs can be stung by the nematocysts, resulting in the condition known as nudibranch dermatitis.

2. It appears that coelenterates may release antigenic and allergenic venom substances in their aquatic environment. Allergens in the venom may sensitize individuals without immediate contact with nematocysts. A severe allergic dermatitis may result if the sensitized individual comes into contact with a ruptured stinging capsule.

Chapter I— References:

1. Russell FE, Carlson RW: Jellyfish stings, in Conn HF (ed): *Current Therapy*. Philadelphia, WB Saunders Co., 1975, pp 872-873.

2. Stillway CW, Lane CE: Phospholipase in the nematocyst toxin of *Physalia physalis*. *Toxicon* 9:193. July 1971.

3. Russell FE: Physalia stings. A report of two cases. *Toxicon* 4:65, 1966.

4. Ioannides G, Davis, JH: Portuguese man-of-war stinging. *Arch Derm* 91:448, May 1965.

5. Arnold HL: Portuguese man-of-war ("bluebottle") stings: Treatment with papain. *Straub Clinic Proc* 37:30, 1971.

6. Marr JJ: Portuguese man-of-war envenomization. *JAMA* 199:337, 1967.

7. Halstead BW: *Poisonous and Venomous Marine Animals of the World. Vol 1*. Invertebrates. Washington, DC, US Government Printing Office, 1965.

8. Mitchell JC: Biochemical basis of geographic ecology. *Int Derm* 14:239, May 1975.

Dermatitis Caused by Echinoderms
(Spiny Creatures)

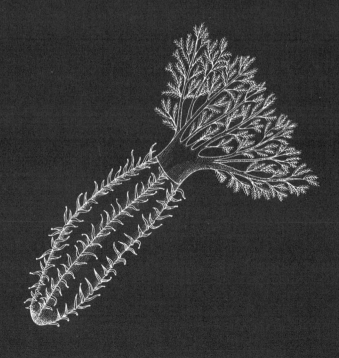

Sea cucumber *Cucumaria*

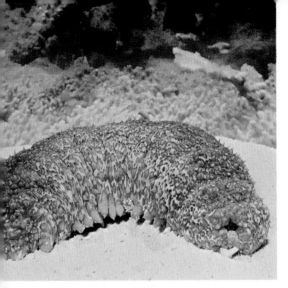

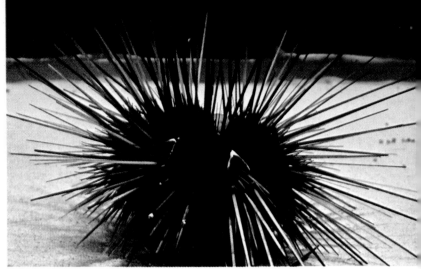

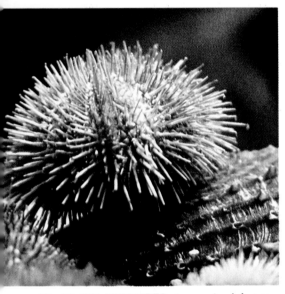

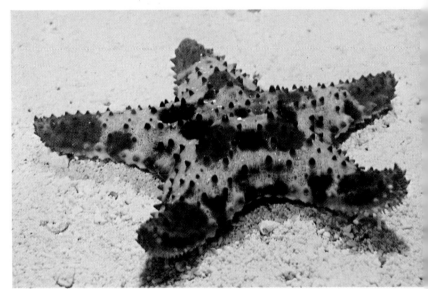

Fig. 2-1. *SEA CUCUMBER.* A sea animal that may occasionally produce a mild dermatitis, the sea cucumber lives in a variety of habitats. It is found from the warm, shallow waters off the coast of Florida, the Bahamas, the Gulf of Mexico, and the Caribbean, to the deeper, colder waters off the coasts of England and Ireland.
Courtesy of the Miami Seaquarium

Fig. 2-3. *GREEN URCHIN.* This member of the sea urchin family shelters itself under coral reefs, rocks or on the sandy or muddy bottoms close to shore. It inhabits the warm waters off the coast of Florida, through the Keys, the Gulf of Mexico and throughout the Caribbean.
Courtesy of the Miami Seaquarium

Fig. 2-2. *SEA URCHIN. Echinodermata diadema* is covered with numerous movable spines which are formed by the calcification of a cylindrical projection of subepidermal connective tissue. These spines are extremely brittle and may break off easily in the victim's skin.
Courtesy of Anthony Healy, M.D.

Fig. 2-4. *STARFISH—CUSHIONED STAR. Coreaster reticulatus* has simple thorny spines of calcium carbonate crystal (calcite) intermingled with organic substances. These spines, held erect by a series of muscles, may produce a papular dermatitis.
Courtesy of the Miami Seaquarium

Dermatitis Caused by Echinoderms
(Spiny Creatures)

With the growing popularity of underwater activities, dermatologists should be on the lookout for echinoderm-caused injuries.

The class Echinoidea, or sea urchins, forms part of the phylum Echinodermata, which also includes starfish and sea cucumbers. The literature on coral reef echinoderms goes back to the earliest phases of sea exploration. Aristotle wrote several notable passages on species of starfishes and sea urchins.

Echinoderms are shy, unaggressive, slow-moving animals who are continually at the mercy of their environment. Unfortunately for humans who come into contact with these creatures, one of the echinoderm's principal means of defense is an array of sharp or toxic spines. There are approximately 6,000 species of echinoderms of which at least 80 are known to be venomous or poisonous.

Injuries from sea urchin spines are a familiar occupational hazard of fishermen in the Mediterranean and many tropical areas. In addition, the growing popularity of underwater activities among vacationers in these regions is presenting many dermatologists with a new diagnostic problem. Awareness of the hazard is the key to proper management.

Sea Urchin Dermatitis

Sea urchins are spherical organisms generally found on the rocky bottoms of salt waters, although some species prefer to burrow in the sand. They are covered with numerous movable spines, the length of which varies with the species. Formed by the calcification of a cylindrical projection of subepidermal connective tissue,[1] these spines are extremely brittle and may break off easily in the victim's skin. The spines of some species are venomous and may contain a neurotoxin.

Sea urchin dermatitis is produced by broken off spines and/or pedicellariae (pincerlike organs), both of which may contain toxic substances.

Intermingled among the spines are pedicellariae—small pincerlike organs or fangs. These organs are attached to stalks that may be shorter or longer than the spines. Venom from the pedicellariae may be injected into the victim's skin via hook-like jaws or valves.

Diagnosis of sea urchin dermatitis is relatively simple if the patient recalls and mentions the original injury. In many cases, however, the immediate reaction may have been so slight that the patient failed to even notice initial contact with the organism. The diagnostician should be aware that some sea urchin spines contain a dye that may discolor the patient's skin and subcutaneous tissues, thereby giving the false impression that the spine is embedded in the skin. The x-ray is diagnostic for the presence of spines.

Two types of sea urchin reactions have been noted:

First aid treatment of sea urchin injury consists of immersing the affected part in water as hot as can be tolerated. Pedicellariae, if present, should be pulled out.

1. *Immediate reactions.* A severe burning pain which may persist for several hours, with or without edema, is the chief immediate symptom of sea urchin dermatitis. Some patients bleed profusely.

Secondary infection may introduce further complications and may be severe when multiple lesions are present. Infected discharging wounds may be a means by which the tissues get rid of infected spines.

Treat painful edematous lesions with water as hot as can be tolerated until the symptoms disappear. Application of an antibiotic is indicated when secondary infection is present. In the absence of secondary infection, lesions usually heal within a week or two providing no portion of the spine remains with the wound.

Certain sea urchin spines are readily phagocytosed in the tissues and dissolve without difficulty. If the spine does not dissolve, surgical removal should be considered. In the acute stage, such removal may be rendered difficult by the fragility of undissolved spines and the presence of dyes which interfere with proper visualization. Removal of spines should not be attempted unless they are easily seen. Visualization via x-ray examination is essential prior to surgical removal.

Strauss and McDonald[2] stress that complications may arise, particularly when spines are embedded over bony prominences within joints, or in contact with nerves. These authors describe a previously unreported case of neuropathy associated with sea urchin injuries. They emphasize that when sea urchin injuries necessitate exploration, aseptic surgical technique is required.

Sea urchin injury may produce an immediate painful wound or a delayed painless granuloma.

2. *Delayed reactions.* After an interval of two or three months following the initial injury, delayed reactions may develop. These reactions may be nodular or diffuse. Lesions of both types are very persistent, and although spontaneous resolution may ultimately occur, it cannot be relied upon as a consistent eventuality.

The nodular form of granulomatous lesion consists of small firm nodules. Some nodules are flesh colored, while others take on the color of the dye in the spines.

Intralesional injections of a corticosteroid are sometimes effective in treating such lesions. If the presence of spines is revealed upon x-ray examination, surgical removal is indicated.

Meneghini[3] reports on a clinical experiment in which he used water-alcohol extracts from the spines of sea urchins. These extracts produced a positive allergic delayed intradermal reaction in two fishermen with sea urchin granulomas. Controls did not develop such reactions (see Table 2-1).

The *diffuse* delayed reaction, occurring mostly in the fingers

Table 2-1

Sea Urchin Spine Experiment*

Patient	Sex	Age (years)	Onset	Evolution	Water–Alcohol	Water†
1	Male	16	6 weeks before	partial recovery with liquid nitrogen	negative	negative
2	Male	14	1 month before	partial recovery with liquid nitrogen	negative	negative
3	Male	20	1 year before	partial recovery with liquid nitrogen	+++ (markedly positive)	+++
4	Male	15	1 month before	recovery	negative	negative
5	Male	28	2 years before	partial recovery	+++	+++
6	Male	30	2 months before	ulceration; very slow recovery	not done	not done

*Meneghini, CL: Cases of sea urchin granuloma with positive intradermal test to spine extracts. *Contact Dermatitis Newsletter, No. 12*, Aug 1972, p. 316.

†Intradermal tests with water-soluble and water-alcohol (filtered) homogenates prepared from spines of sea urchins of the Echinus family.

and toes, takes the form of a cyanotic induration. Swelling may produce a fusiform deformity. In severe cases, the phalanges may show focal destruction with joint involvement. Combined systemic antibiotic and corticosteroid chemotherapy is the recommended treatment in such patients.

Histologic changes associated with sea urchin lesions show a wide range of variation. There may be microabscesses or a chronic granulomatous inflammatory reaction of foreign-body type,[4] and double refractable particles may sometimes be detected.[5] However, the histology of the skeletal granulomas may give no clue as to their origin.[6]

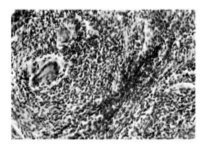

Fig. 2-5. *SEA URCHIN GRANULOMA — HISTOLOGY.* Biopsy of a sea urchin granuloma reveals a lesion packed with lymphocytes. Some of these have a central necrotic area with polynuclear cells.
Courtesy of William Orris, M.D.

Starfish Dermatitis

Starfishes have simple thorny spines of calcium carbonate crystal (calcite) intermingled with organic substances. The spines are held erect by a number of muscles. Specialized glandular tissue embedded in the calcite is capable of secreting a toxin which can be discharged into the water or perhaps directly into the skin.

The toxic substance exuded by the starfish is apparently diffusible in water and alcohol. Consequently, when large numbers of starfish are present, contact with the surrounding water may produce a pruritic papulourticarial eruption. Calamine lotion with 0.5% menthol is a soothing preparation for such dermatitis.

In addition, the starfish *Acanthaster planci* ("crown of thorns") can inflict a painful sting when its venomous aboral spines pierce the skin. Such injury may produce granulomatous lesions requiring surgical excision.

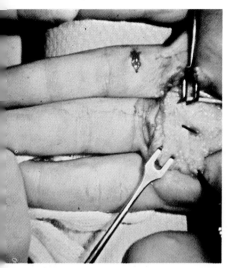

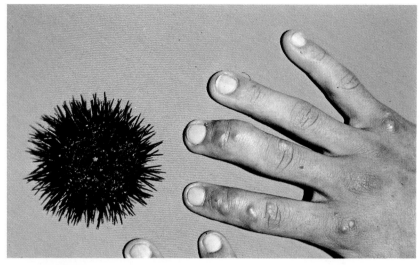

Fig. 2-6. *SEA URCHIN INJURY* is caused by the pedicellariae which can break off in the skin when the animal is pulled off. One of these pedicellariae is shown in a patient's hand.
Courtesy of Bruce W. Halstead, M.D. and Maurice B. Strauss, M.D.

Fig. 2-7. *SEA URCHIN GRANULOMA.* Multiple granulomas caused by a sea urchin injury are seen on the hands and fingers of this patient.
Courtesy of A.H. Menghini, M.D.

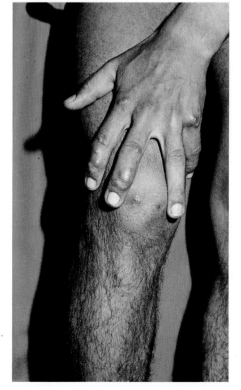

Fig. 2-8. *SEA URCHIN GRANULOMA.* After an interval of two or three months following the initial injury, delayed reactions may develop. These may be nodular or diffuse. In this instance, the reactions are nodular.

Sea Cucumber Dermatitis

The visceral liquid ejected by the animal sea cucumbers *Cucumaria* and *Stichopus* can cause irritation of the skin and the eyes.[7] The skin manifestation is a papular eruption caused by the toxic material holothurin, which is produced in the body wall of the sea cucumber. Holothurin consists of cardiac glycosides or steroid saponins,[8] such as have been previously identified in plants.

In a personal communication to W. L. Orris, M.D., formerly Director of Medical Services, Scripps Institution of Oceanography, University of California, San Diego, A. H. Banner, Professor of Zoology at the University of Hawaii, reported that "when my children were small they took delight in throwing apodous holothurian, *Opheodesoma spectabilis,* at each other. I had finally to forbid it because it caused a skin rash; whether it was from the anchor-shaped spicules or from toxic compounds, I do not know."

Some sea cucumbers feed on the nematocysts of coelenterates and retain the stinging nematocyst apparatus in an intact state for use in their own defense. The clinician should be aware of this possibility in managing skin reactions resulting from contact with sea cucumbers. The application of alcohol to skin that has come in contact with such sea cucumbers will detoxify any nematocysts present (see Chapter I).

The sea cucumber exudes holothurin, a toxin which can produce papular urticaria, conjunctivitis and blindness. This echinoderm may also feed on nematocysts and use such cysts for its own defense.

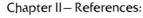

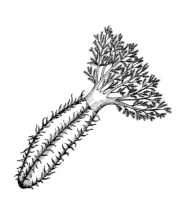

Chapter II — References:

1. Nicholas D: *Echinoderms*. London, Hutchinson, 1962.

2. Strauss MB, McDonald RI: Hand injuries from sea urchins. *Clin Orthop 114*:216, 1976.

3. Meneghini CL: Cases of sea urchin granuloma with positive intradermal test to spine extracts. *Contact Dermatitis Newsletter, No. 12*, Aug. 1972, p. 316.

4. O'Neal RL, *et al.*: Injury to human tissues from sea urchin stings. *Calif Med 101*:199, 1964.

5. Rocha G, Fraga S: Sea urchin granuloma of the skin. *Arch Derm 85*:406, 1962.

6. Mortensen T: *A monograph of the Echinoidea*. Index to Vols. I-V. Carlsberg-Fund, C.A. Reitzel, Copenhagen. 1951, 63 pp.

7. Halstead BW: *Poisonous and venomous marine animals of the world. Vol. 1.* Invertebrates. Washington, D.C., US Government Printing Office, 1965, pp. 537-580.

8. Rothberg I, *et al.*: Terpenoids. LXVIII. 23-epsilon-acetoxy-17—deoxy-7, 8-dihydro-holothurinogen, a new triteripenoid sapogenin from a sea cucumber. *J Org Chem 38*:209, 1973.

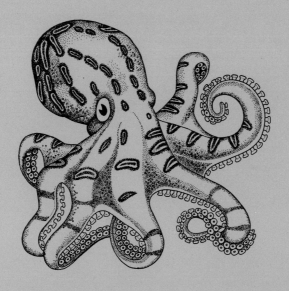

Spotted octopus *Octopusus maculosus*

Eruptions and Reactions
Caused by Mollusks

The phylum Mollusca consists of unsegmented, soft-bodied invertebrates, most of which secrete calcareous shells. Mollusks respire by means of gills or a modified primitive pulmonary sac; some species are equipped with jaws.

It has been estimated that 45,000 species of mollusks inhabit the waters of the globe, probably constituting the largest single group of biotoxic marine invertebrates of direct importance to man. Within the phylum Mollusca, the pelecypods (scallops, oysters, clams, etc.) appear to cause the greatest number of human intoxications annually. The next most important group in terms of biotoxicity are the gastropods (snails, slugs), with the cephalopods (squid, octopus, cuttlefish, etc.) ranking third.[1]

Only two classes—Gastropoda and Cephalopoda—have been definitely implicated in the precipitation of dermatologic reactions.

Gastropods (snails, slugs) and cephalopods (squid, octopus) are the marine organisms of the mollusk family most capable of producing dermatoses.

Cone Shells

The most dangerous members of the class Gastropoda are of the genus *Conus*, family Conidae. Many tropical and subtropical species —notably *Conus aulicus, C. geographus, C. gloria-maris, C. marmoreus, C. omaria, C. striatus, C. textile,* and *C. tulipa* —have a venom apparatus well developed enough to inflict human fatalities. A 15% to 20% mortality rate has been reported for some of the more deadly of these gastropods found in Australia and California.[2] Off the Florida coast, species such as the Chinese alphabet cone, *C. spurius* Auct, and the queen cone, *C. regius* Chemnitz, have been suspected of being dangerous.[3]

Because of the attractiveness of the shells, Conidae is avidly sought after for private and public collections. Hence, its main victims are careless collectors who have not taken proper precautions.

These potentially deadly creatures are small, usually only about four inches in length. They are for the most part shallow-water inhabitants. Some species are found in the attached algae of coral reefs; others crawl in the vicinity of coral heads; still others feel most at home in a sandy or coral rubble substrate. Species most hazardous to man are those which inhabit the sand or rubble. Cone shells are nocturnal creatures; they burrow in the sand or coral in the daytime, and emerge to feed at night on a varied fare

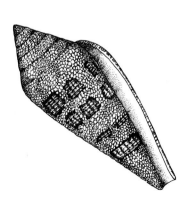

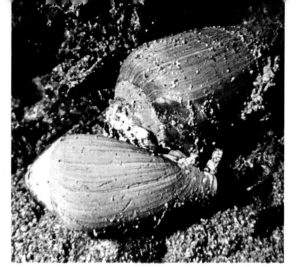

Fig. 3-1. *CONE SHELLS.* Small, but potentially deadly, cone shells are usually only about four inches in length. They inflict their stings by means of venomous rasping teeth which lie dormant in a radular sheath when not in use.
Courtesy of Michael D. Rosco, M.D.

A particularly dangerous mollusk is the venomous Conus. This creature can inflict painful puncture wounds with local ischemia, cyanosis and numbness spreading to involve the entire body. The sting may be fatal.

that includes other gastropods, as well as octopuses, pelecypods, and small fishes.

Envenomization Mechanism. Cone shells inflict their stings by means of venomous radular (rasping) teeth which lie dormant in a sheath when not in use. When needed, a single tooth passes from the sheath through the pharynx, where it is charged with venom produced in the venom duct.[4] The tooth then passes from the pharynx into the anterior opening of the proboscis and is there held ready to pierce the hapless victim. The chemistry and pharmacology of cone shell venom have yet to be clearly elucidated; there is some evidence that cone shell venoms vary from one species to the next.[4]

Dermatologic Symptoms. Cone shell stings are of the puncture-wound variety. Initial symptoms generally include a sharp stinging or burning sensation, or localized ischemia, cyanosis, and numbness in the area of the wound. Pain varies from one patient to the next. One patient will complain that the pain is excruciating, while another will report that it is no greater than an insect sting. Generalized pruritus may be a problem in some patients.

Systemic Symptoms. Numbness, swelling, and paresthesia beginning at the wound site may spread rapidly and involve the entire body, particularly the lips and mouth. In severe cases, early paralysis of the voluntary muscles may be followed by a complete generalized muscular paralysis. Aphonia and dysphagia, if present,

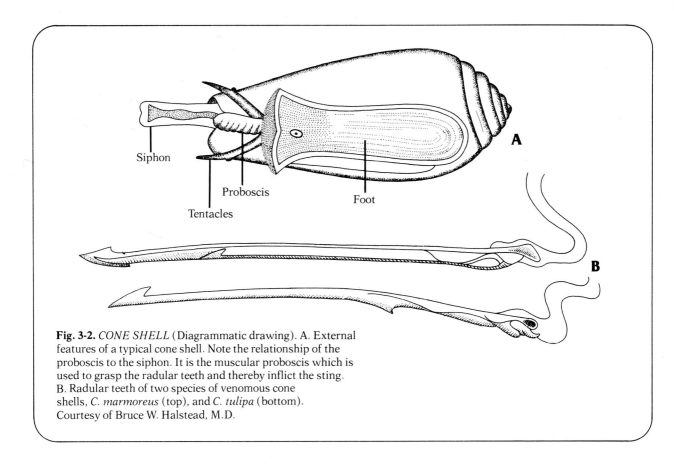

Fig. 3-2. *CONE SHELL* (Diagrammatic drawing). A. External features of a typical cone shell. Note the relationship of the proboscis to the siphon. It is the muscular proboscis which is used to grasp the radular teeth and thereby inflict the sting. B. Radular teeth of two species of venomous cone shells, *C. marmoreus* (top), and *C. tulipa* (bottom). Courtesy of Bruce W. Halstead, M.D.

Siphon

Proboscis

Tentacles

Foot

A

B

may be marked and cause the victim great distress. Blurred vision and diplopia are common symptoms. Gastrointestinal symptoms, with the exception of nausea, are usually absent. Coma and cardiac failure may ensue.

Though treatment of cone shell stings is empiric, syringing with strong soap solution, heat treatments and use of neostygmine have been suggested.

Treatment. Treatment of cone shell stings is entirely empiric and symptomatic. Although local measures are usually of little value, syringing the wound with a strong soap solution should be attempted. Heat treatments have been reported to be useful.[2] Although cone shells do not produce a typical curare-like blocking agent, the use of neostigmine has been suggested.[1] In severe stings, maintenance of circulating blood volume with intravenous solutions and vasopressor agents may be essential. Local injection of epinephrine has been recommended, but its value remains unproven.[5]

Preventive Measures. Collectors who fancy cone shells should always wear gloves. The animal should be picked up by the large posterior end of the shell, and should be dropped immediately if the proboscis is extended from the pointed anterior end. Cone shells should never be held in the hand any longer than necessary. Most stings have occurred while the collector was attempting to scrape encrusted organic debris from the shell. Possibly, the scraping process stimulates the cone to strike.[1]

Sea Butterflies

Pteropods, or sea butterflies, are small gastropods rarely exceeding an inch in length. Although they are found in abundance in open seas throughout the world, biologic data about sea butterflies are scarce. Briefly, what is known about them is that they are hermaphroditic and that they feed essentially on protozoans and microscopic algae. There is a total of some 60 species.

Pteropod stings evoke a maculopapular rash resembling that produced by certain coelenterates. However, unlike the dermatologic sequelae associated with coelenterates, sea butterfly stings do not appear to elicit serious dermatologic manifestations following the initial sting.

An outbreak of stingings, presumably caused by the straight-needle pteropod *Creseis acicula,* was reported off St. Petersburg, Florida.[1] The stings were believed to have occurred when these needle-like gastropods penetrated swimmers' bathing suits. Whether the lesions resulted from the mechanical effects of contact or from a toxic substance has never been established.

Treatment, when necessary, is entirely symptomatic.

Octopuses and Other Cephalopods

Few marine creatures have received as much popular attention as the octopus, a member of the Cephalopoda class of mollusks which also includes squids and cuttlefish. Despite the fabled reputation of "giant octopuses" which threaten ships and attack divers, octopuses and squids are generally harmless and retiring; few are be-

The large octopuses are usually harmless. However, the tiny blue-ringed octopus can inflict a fatal bite.

lieved to be venomous.[2] The chief exception, ironically, appears to be the tiny *Hapalochlaena maculosa* or blue-ringed octopus—only three to four inches long, and found mainly in Australian coastal waters. It has been called the world's most deadly octopus—even more deadly, according to Dr. J. Trinka, Deputy Director of the Commonwealth Serum Laboratories of Australia, than Australian snakes, which are considered the world's most lethal.[6] Some experts have reported a 25% mortality rate following bites by the blue-ringed octopus.[2] Normally *H. maculosa* is a rather inconspicuous creature, but when threatened or angered the bluish patterns on its predominantly yellowish brown body and arms become an irridescent peacock blue. These bright colors often attract bathers and divers.

Human fatalities and near fatalities seem to follow a fairly identical pattern.[7] The octopus, found stranded in a rock pool, is placed on the back of the hand or arm and displayed to interested

Fig. 3-3. *OCTOPUS BITE.* A subungual hemorrhage and laceration of a finger characterizes octopus bites. In this instance, a young boy picked up a tin can while exploring the tidal pools at La Jolla, California. The octopus hidden in the can bit him when he attempted to pull it off his finger. The bite usually manifests as two small puncture wounds produced by the sharp, parrot-like jaws of the cephalopod.
Courtesy of William Orris, M.D.

Fig. 3-4. *BLUE-RINGED OCTOPUS.* Only three to four inches long, this small creature is found mainly in Australian coastal waters. It is probably the world's most deadly octopus. Normally it is a rather inconspicuous creature, but when threatened or angered the bluish patterns on its yellowish brown body and arms become an irridescent peacock blue.
Courtesy of Michael D. Rosco, M.D.

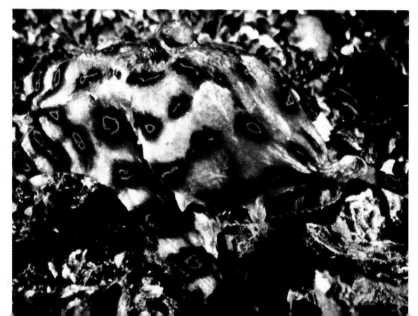

Symptoms arising from the puncture-like bite may include pain, profuse bleeding, intense pruritus, plus numerous systemic manifestations. Immediate excision of the wound is recommended.

Fig. 3-5. *ENVENOMATING MECH-ANISM OF RINGED OCTOPUS* (*H. maculosa*). Venom-containing saliva passes through salivary duct into buccal mass and finally into wound inflicted by beak and rasp-like tongue (not indicated).

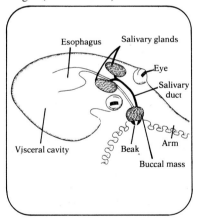

Esophagus Salivary glands
Eye
Salivary duct
Visceral cavity Beak
Arm
Buccal mass

parties, or carried to the beach. Frequently the victim is unaware of any actual bite, but symptoms occur within five or ten minutes.

Symptoms. The bite usually manifests as two small puncture wounds produced by the sharp, parrot-like jaws of the cephalopod. Pain, when immediately present, is a burning and stinging sensation; some patients describe it as similar to that of a bee sting. Initially localized, the pain may radiate to include the entire appendage. Within a few minutes, a tingling or pulsating sensation develops in the area of the wound. The profuse and prolonged bleeding characteristic of these stings suggests that coagulation time is retarded. Swelling, redness, and heat generally develop around the wound and some victims complain of an intense pruritus.[4] Allergic urticarial reaction has also been reported.[8]

In severe cases, systemic symptoms may include numbness of the mouth and tongue, blurring of vision, difficulty in speech and swallowing, loss of tactile sensation and equilibrium and muscular paralysis. Death, when it occurs, appears to be associated with respiratory failure.

Treatment. Rosco[2] reports that there is no effective treatment other than immediate excision of the wound. He recommends a circular skin incision, removal of all the subcutaneous tissue down to the deep fascia, then reapplication of the skin on the wound as a full thickness free graft.[2]

No antivenin against the blue-ringed octopus is yet available, but research toward this end is being conducted at the Commonwealth Serum Laboratories in Parkville, Victoria, Australia.

Map 3-1.
**Distribution of Reported
Cone Shell Stings**

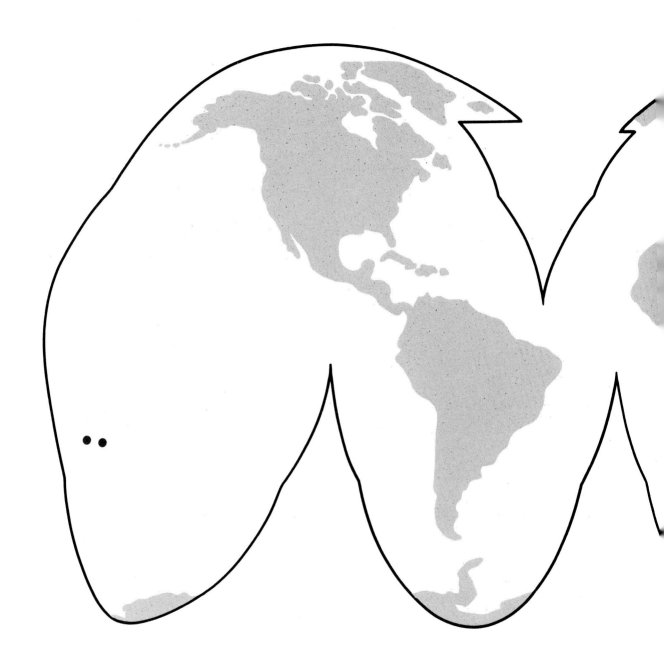

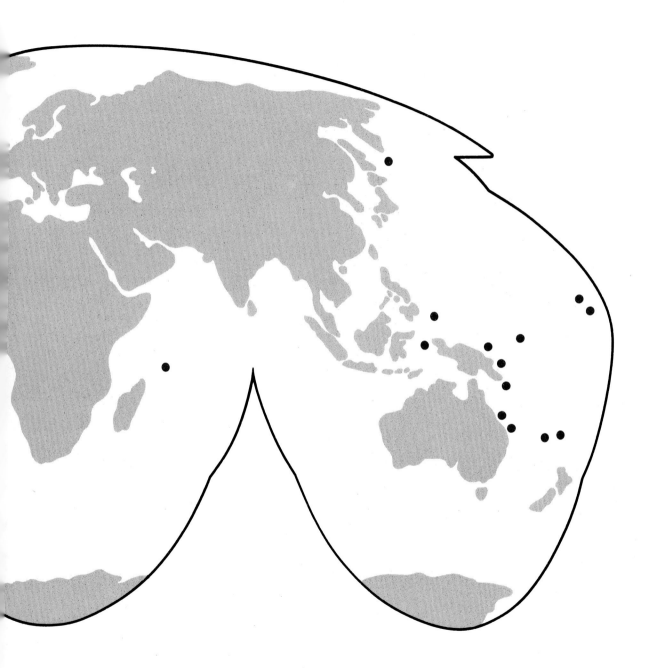

(Adapted from Halstead BW: Poisonous and Venomous Marine Animals of the World. Vol. 1. Washington, DC, US Government Printing Office, 1965, p 880.)

Chapter III—References:

1. Halstead BW: *Poisonous and Venomous Marine Animals of the World. Vol 1. Invertebrates.* Washington, DC, US Government Printing Office, 1965.

2. Rosco D: Treatment of venomous and poisonous marine animal injuries. *Int'l Soc Aquatic Med Newsletter,* Vol 2, No. 2, June 1976.

3. Phillips C, Brady WH: *Sea Pests—Poisonous or Harmful Sea Life of Florida and the West Indies.* Miami, Univ. Miami Press, 1953.

4. Halstead BW: Marine biotoxicology, in Coulston F (ed): *EQS Environmental Quality and Safety, Vol 3.* New York, Academic Press.

5. Russell F: Animal venoms, in *Practice of Medicine, Vol 9.* Hagerstown, Md, Harper & Row Publishers, Inc, 1975.

6. Deas W: Venomous octopus. *Sea Frontiers (Magazine of the International Oceanographic Foundation) 16*:357, Nov-Dec 1970.

7. Sutherland SK, Lane WR: Toxins and mode of envenomation of the common ringed or blue-banded octopus. *Med J Aust 1*:893, May 3, 1969.

8. Edmonds C: A non-fatal case of blue-ringed octopus bite. *Med J Aust 2*:601, Sept 20, 1969.

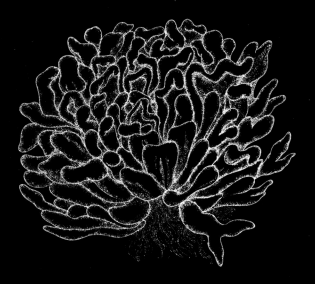

Red beard sponge *Microciona prolifera*

Dermatitis Caused by Sponges

Sponges are stationary animals living attached to the sea bottom. Our familiar bath sponges are in fact the skeletons of certain Porifera which inhabit warm waters. These skeletons are composed of spongin, a fibrous material that retains its elastic properties long after the sponge is dead. Sponges were recorded as plants for many centuries but received animal status from zoologists in 1835.[1] Mitchell[2] reports that in a current textbook on dermatology, a paper on a skin reaction from the sponge, *Tedania ignis,* is erroneously listed under dermatitis from plants. Both freshwater animal sponges and marine animal sponges can cause contact dermatitis.

Fire Sponge Dermatitis

Tedania ignis, also known as "fire sponge," is abundant in the Miami area and near the shore along the Florida Keys. The nickname is appropriate when one considers both the fire sponge's color and its stinging apparatus. The color is normally a brilliant vermilion or reddish orange, although orange or yellowish orange fire sponges are occasionally seen. The sponge grows as a bunch of branches or "fingers" extending upward from a main base. Despite its stinging powers, it usually harbors a host of marine worms, shrimps, and other small crustacea which live unharmed in the central cavity.

The fire sponge has no commercial value but is nonetheless a beautiful creature.

If detached, or particularly if one of the "fingers" is broken, the fire sponge is capable of producing a dermatitis resembling that of poison ivy. The patient initially experiences an itching or prickling sensation, followed in a few hours by swelling, stiffness, and considerable discomfort. If the fingers are stung, they become immovable within a day; any attempt to flex them is accompanied by pain. Symptoms usually subside within two days, when there is a gradual reduction of swelling and return of normal movement in the affected area.

Treatment of fire sponge dermatitis is the same as for severe poison ivy dermatitis.

In addition to the just described skin reaction, fire sponge can also produce an erythema multiforme type of eruption. This reaction has been attributed to a pharmacologically active substance which may also be a sensitizer.

Both freshwater and marine sponges may produce a severe irritant chemical dermatitis with marked edema.

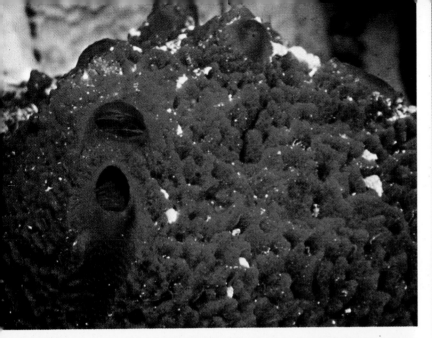

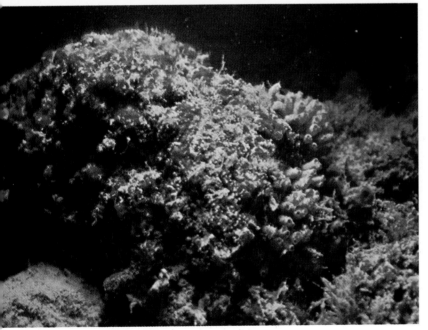

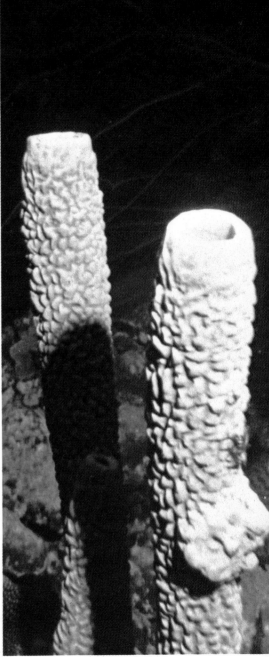

Fig. 4-1. *FIRE SPONGE. Tedania ignis* is usually a brilliant red-orange, although some may be yellow-orange. This sponge is abundant in the Miami area and near the shore along the Florida Keys.

Fig. 4-2. *FIRE SPONGE* grows as a bunch of branches or "fingers" extending upward from a main base. If the fingers are broken or detached, the fire sponge is capable of producing a dermatitis resembling poison ivy. Courtesy of Bruce W. Halstead, M.D.

Fig. 4-3. *SPONGE SKELETONS* are composed of spongin, a fibrous material that retains its elastic properties long after the sponge is dead. Both freshwater animal sponges and marine animal sponges can cause contact dermatitis. Courtesy of Michael D. Rosco, M.D.

47

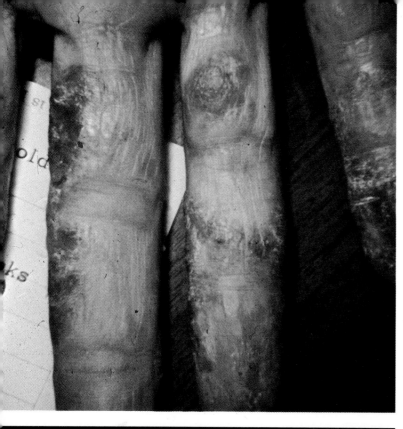

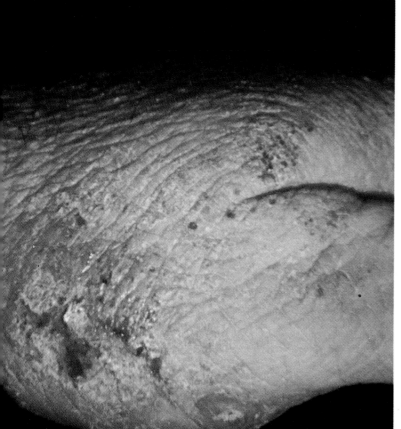

Fig. 4-4 *FIRE SPONGE DERMATITIS* of the fingers produced marked stiffness and immobility within a day. Any attempt to flex the fingers was accompanied by pain.
Courtesy of William Orris, M.D.

Fig. 4-5. *FIRE SPONGE ERUPTION* typically becomes eczematous and crusted, as shown here.

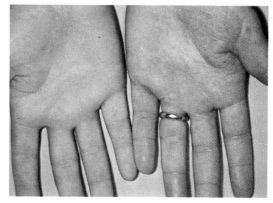

Fig. 4-6. *FIRE SPONGE DERMATITIS.* The patient initially experienced an itching, prickling sensation. This was followed in a few hours by swelling, stiffness and aching pain.
Courtesy of Wiley M. Sams, M.D.

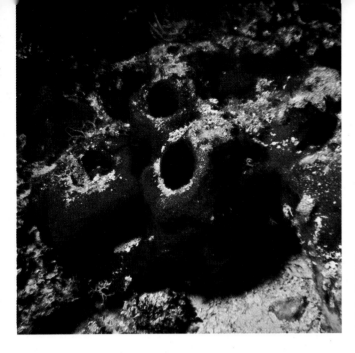

Fig. 4-7. *POISON BUN SPONGE,*
Neofibularia nolitangere. Photo, taken
on the barrier reef of Belize (Central
America), near Carrie Bow Cay, covers
an area approximately one square foot.
Courtesy of K. Ruetzler

Poison Bun Sponge Dermatitis

Less common than *Tedania,* the "poison bun sponge," *Fibula
nolitangere,* ranges into somewhat deeper water. The appellation
"nolitangere" ("do not touch") is appropriate: *Fibula's* sting is
reported to produce an even more violent reaction than that of the
fire sponge.

The poison bun sponge is relatively difficult to recognize, since
it closely resembles a number of other common sponges in size,
shape, and color. It generally grows in small masses, occasionally
in small lumps, and the oscula (holes) are usually large enough to
admit a finger. *Fibula* is brownish on the outside and drab on
the inside with a soft "bready" texture. The skin is exposed to the
toxic substance when one contacts the surface of this sponge or
breaks it.

Treatment is the same as for severe poison ivy dermatitis.

Red Sponge Dermatitis

The red sponge, *Microciona prolifera,* may produce erythema and
edema of the hands and stiffness of the joints in oyster fishermen
and others who handle it. Subsequently, bullae develop and may
become purulent. If not properly treated, the eruption may persist
for several months.

A patch test with a small piece of sponge confirms the diagnosis.
The treatment is the same as for severe poison ivy dermatitis.

Sponge Spicule Dermatitis

In addition to the stinging sponges, which produce dermatitis via chemical action, some sponges can cause traumatic injuries. Certain sponges are equipped with a skeletal matrix containing silicon dioxide spicules or calcium carbonate spicules. Both types may produce an irritation when broken off in the skin, and both are difficult to remove once they have penetrated.

The application of adhesive tape to the affected area is sometimes efficacious, since the spicules may adhere to the tape. Isopropyl alcohol should be applied after the adhesive tape is removed.

Patients should be advised to wear canvas gloves when handling living sponges that can cause injuries.

> Some sponge may trigger a foreign body reaction due to penetration of the skin with sponge spicules. Application of adhesive tape is often an effective method of removal.

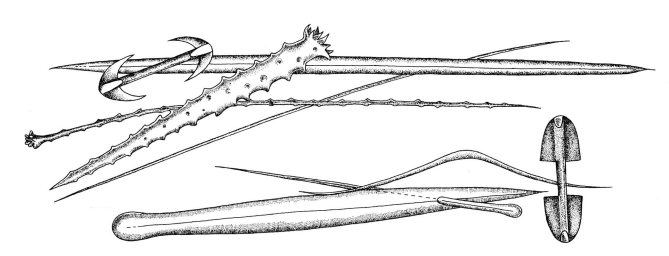

Fig. 4-8. *DIFFERENT FORMS OF SPONGE SPICULES.*

CHAPTER IV—References:

1. Halstead BW: *Poisonous and Venomous Marine Animals of the World. Vol. 1.* Invertebrates. Washington, DC, US Government Printing Office, 1965.
2. Mitchell JC: Biochemical basis of geographic ecology. *Int Derm 14:*239, May 1975.

V

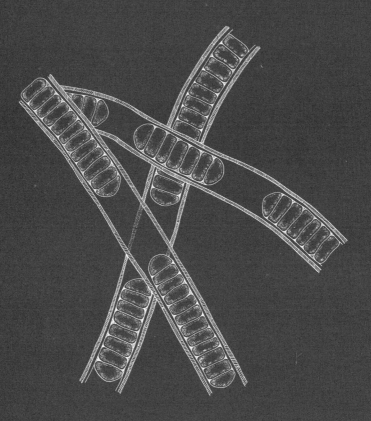

Alga *Lyngbya majuscula*

Dermatitis Caused by Seaweed

The two types of seaweed dermatitis are the animal plant variety, including sea moss or sea mat dermatitis ("Dogger Bank itch"), and the marine plant variety, including Hawaiian dermatitis due to algea.

Seaweed Dermatitis Due to Algae

Approximately 30,000 species of algae have been identified. Although they are included among the lowest divisions of the vegtable kingdom and most contain chlorophyll, many algae are equipped with flagella and propel themselves through the water very much like animals.[1] Algae grow in a variety of sizes, shapes, and colors. The smallest are microscopic, such as the snowflake-like diatoms which are barely a micron in diameter. The giant kelp, which may attain a length of 300 feet, is among the largest algae.

One of the plant kingdom's most ubiquitous members, algae may be found in almost every type of environment. Primitive blue-green algae thrive in the water of hot springs that attain a temperature of 160°F; others may be found in freshwater, salt water, and in the snow, ice, and waters of the Arctic regions.[2] Some are saprophytic or symbiotic—growing in or on other plants and animals. Viable, growing algae have been found at ocean depths of 12,000 feet, despite the fact that sunlight can only penetrate ocean waters to a depth of 900 feet. The means by which they accomplish this is still a matter of conjecture among scientists.

The algae of medical importance to the dermatologist are those found in running waters, ponds, lakes, and oceans. These consist mainly of the blue-green alga, *Lyngbya majuscula*. *Lyngbya* looks somewhat like hair. Not all strains are toxic. One area may have a toxic strain, while the algae may be nontoxic just a few miles away.[3] *Lyngbya* occurs in abundance from the intertidal zone to a depth of 100 feet—representing a hazard to sensitized swimmers.

Grauer and Arnold[3] reported 125 cases of seaweed dermatitis treated in Hawaii following contact with *Lyngbya*. Hundreds of other mild, unreported cases were suspected. As can be seen on the map (page 53), the cases occurred at beaches from Laie and Kaaawa to Lanikai—and possibly Waimanalo—with no instances of occurrence in Kaneohe Bay. (Later, Hawaiian dermatologists saw similar cases where the alga was encountered on the wind-

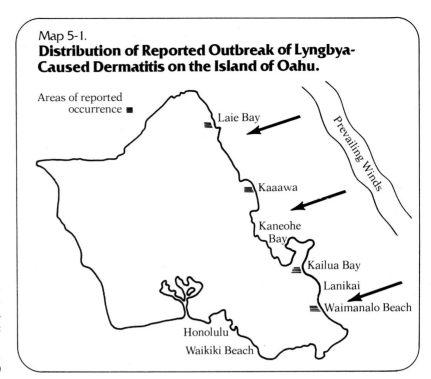

Map 5-1.
Distribution of Reported Outbreak of Lyngbya-Caused Dermatitis on the Island of Oahu.

Areas of reported occurrence ≡

Laie Bay

Prevailing Winds

Kaaawa

Kaneohe Bay

Kailua Bay

Lanikai

Waimanalo Beach

Honolulu

Waikiki Beach

Note that sites of dermatitis were on the windward shore. It was thought that the alga may have come from the open sea since no cases were reported at protected Kaneohe Bay. (Adapted from Grauer FH, Arnold HL: Seaweed dermatitis. Arch Derm *84*:720, Nov 1961. © 1961, American Medical Association.)

ward beaches.) The following pattern emerged during this epidemic of *Lyngbya* dermatitis.[3]

• The patient had been swimming, often in water made turbid by suspended fragments of seaweed.

• He or she continued to wear the wet bathing garment after leaving the ocean and before showering.

• A gradual onset of itching and burning occurred within a few minutes to a few hours after emerging from the ocean.

• Visible dermatitis beginning with redness appeared after three to eight hours.

So-called "seaweed dermatitis" due to toxic algae usually affects parts of the body covered by bathing suits.

The initial symptoms are followed by blisters and deep desquamation, leaving a moist, bright red, tender, and painful area on the scrotum, perineum, or perianal region. The eruption appears on the area of the body covered by the bathing suit; male patients are especially affected on the most dependent part of the scrotum. Women patients, especially those wearing close fitting brassieres, are occasionally affected on the breasts.

A few instances of skin reactions to freshwater blue-green algae have also been reported.[4,5]

A number of similarities between seaweed dermatitis and sea-bathers' eruption have been noted (see Chapter VI). Both eruptions occur in the same body region after swimming in salt water at a time when an unusually large amount of seaweed is found on the beaches or in the water. The disorders have a seasonal incidence, occurring in the spring and summer (March-September in Florida and June-September in Hawaii). Finally, both are characterized by a pruritic eruption ensuing within a few hours after swimming, persisting for a few days, and subsiding spontaneously. Obviously, therefore, differential diagnosis between the two conditions may be necessary.

Severe algae dermatitis may require systemic corticosteroids. The most effective measures, however, are prophylactic. The clinician would do well to advise patients who may be swimming in algae-abundant areas to shower with soap and water and wash their bathing suits *immediately* after their swim. Cleaning the beach of accumulated seaweed is also helpful.

Sea Moss Dermatitis
("Dogger Bank itch")

The term "Dogger Bank itch" is usually applied to the eczematous dermatitis caused by the sea-chervil, *Alcyondium hirsutum,* a sea-weed-like animal colony. These sea mosses or sea mats are found on the Dogger Bank—an immense shelf-like elevation under the North Sea between Scotland and Denmark.

North Sea fishermen—particularly those fishing the Dogger Bank area—come into contact with the sea-chervil when it is drawn up in their fishing nets together with the fish. Large quantities of sea-chervil are sometimes landed, then thrown back into the sea.

The dermatitis, first noticed on the hands, clears when the fisherman goes ashore. However, on returning to fishing, increasingly severe attacks may develop, characterized by a blistered and edematous eruption on the hands and arms, face and legs.

Noting that Dogger Bank itch is prevalent among Lowestoft trawlermen, Newhouse[6] describes Dogger Bank itch as an allergic dermatitis resulting from contact with *Alcyonidium* when it is

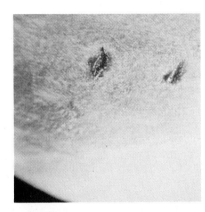

Fig. 5-1. *LYNGBYA LESIONS* produced experimentally on the skin of a guinea pig 24 hours after a subcutaneous injection of toxic Lyngbya emulsion.
Courtesy of George W. Chu, Sc.D.

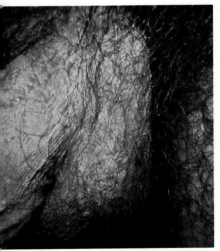

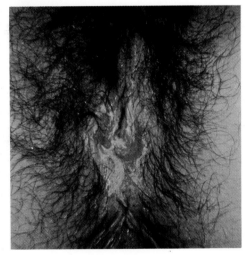

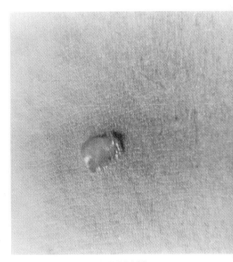

Fig. 5-2. *SEAWEED BURN* of the scrotum produced by contact with Lyngbya. Note the typical shallow burn-like erosion of the scrotum. This type of "burn" is seen in patients who continue to wear wet bathing garments after leaving the ocean and before showering.
Courtesy of
H.L. Arnold, Jr., M.D.

Fig. 5-3. *SEAWEED BURN* of the vulva caused by Lyngba contact. The patient experienced a gradual onset of itching and burning within a few minutes after swimming. This was followed in three to eight hours by blistering and superficial ulceration. Note a typical patch of escharotic dermatitis of the vulva.
Courtesy of
H. L. Arnold, Jr., M.D.

Fig. 5-4. *LYNGBYA DERMATITIS.* Vesiculation produced by the toxic Lyngbya in contact with the contributor's arm after a period of several hours.
Courtesy of
George W. Chu, Sc.D.

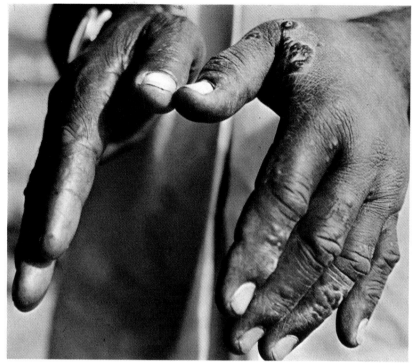

Fig. 5-5. *ALGA DERMATITIS* produced by *Stephanocyphus racemosis* (also called *Nausithoe punctata*). This dermatitis is characterized by marked edema of the hands with bullae and crusting. Another "juvenile" form of the alga is called "stinging alga."
Courtesy of Bruce W. Halstead, M.D.

hauled aboard the vessel with other contents of the trawl. Positive patch test reactions with an extract from the causative marine animals and negative reactions in controls would certainly seem to point to an allergic mechanism. On the other hand, the fact that in many instances all on board acquire dermatitis except the cook (who does not appear on deck) would indicate that an irritant mechanism is operative rather than an allergic reaction.

The condition should be treated in the same manner as a mild poison ivy dermatitis. Calamine lotion is used, as well as 20% alcohol. The alcohol acts as a cooling agent.

Proper protective clothing usually prevents occurrence of the eruption.

Red Moss Dermatitis

Although the animal named red moss *(Microciona)* has been reported to cause a contact reaction on the hands of fisherman, anemones living on the moss actually may be responsible.

Skin reactions attributed to plant moss *(Iosthecium)* are probably caused by contamination of the moss by allergenic chemical compounds of the liverwort plant *(Frullania)*, which grows among the moss.[8]

Treatment is the same as for Dogger Bank itch.

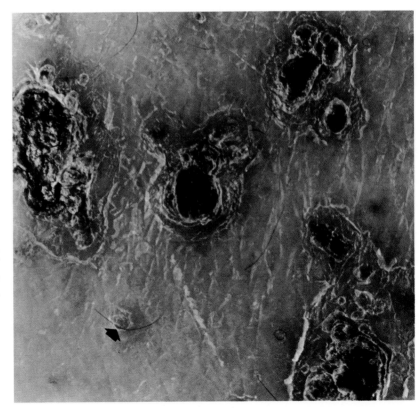

Fig. 5-6. *ACHLORIC INFECTIOUS DERMATITIS.* The crusted ulcerated lesions are surrounded by a zone of erythema. The arrow points to an early papular lesion with little inflammation. Courtesy of John P. Tindall, M.D. and Bernard F. Fetter, M.D.

Chapter V—References:

1. Tiffany HL: *Algae, the Grass of Many Waters.* Springfield, Ill, Charles C. Thomas, 1968.
2. Kavaler L: *The Wonders of Algae.* New York, The John Day Co, 1961.
3. Grauer FH, Arnold HL: Seaweed dermatitis. *Arch Derm 84*:720, Nov 1961.
4. Cohen SG, Reif CB: Cutaneous sensitization to blue-green algae. *J Allergy 24*:452, 1953.
5. Heise HA: II. Microcystis: Another form of algae producing allergenic reactions. *Ann Allergy 9*:100, 1951.
6. Newhouse ML: Dogger Bank itch: Survey of trawlermen. *Rehabilitation 60*:941, 1967.
7. Corson EF, Pratt AG: "Red moss" dermatitis. *Arch Derm Syph 47*:574, 1943.
8. Mitchell JC: Biochemical basis of geographic ecology. *Int Derm 14*:239, May 1975.

Dermatitis Caused by Schistosomes and Other Marine Worms

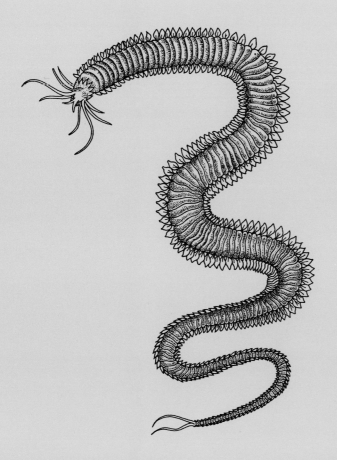

Bristle worm *Nereis virens*

Dermatitis Caused by Schistosomes and Other Marine Worms

Cercarial dermatitis is an infestation resulting from penetration of the skin by the cercariae of schistosomes. These schistosomes are parasitic flatworms having one or more external suckers. Their cercariae—an immature larval form—are usually microscopic in size and are provided with tails.

Schistosome cercarial dermatitis is sometimes referred to as a "disease of the place," exemplifying the widespread geographic distribution of the condition. Reports of schistosome cercarial dermatitis have come from virtually every area of the globe—Occident, Orient, Arctic, temperate and tropical zones, in both fresh and salt water.

According to world health officials, schistosomal infestation—including the dermatitis-producing type—now rivals malaria as the world's number one health problem. In western Africa, the Orient, and the West Indies, many agricultural workers are endangered by this infestation while working in irrigation waters. Swimming and diving activities have become a serious hazard in infested streams or lakes.

Although serious schistosomal infestation is not common in North America, cercarial dermatitis has become a vexing problem on certain freshwater and even saltwater beaches. Snails and birds inhabiting the lake areas of Wisconsin, Michigan, Manitoba, and neighboring North Central states are the intermediate hosts for the infestation.

Terminology

The discussion of schistosome cercarial dermatitis is cluttered by various synonyms that are sometimes used interchangeably: "clam-diggers' itch," "swimmers' itch," and "sea bathers' eruption." Some observers have insisted on a distinction between "swimmers' itch" and "sea bathers' eruption," limiting "swimmers' itch" to the eruption on exposed areas and "sea bathers' eruption" to a dermatitis resulting from ocean bathing.

In my view, these distinctions are artificial and confusing. It is more appropriate to speak of *schistosome cercarial dermatitis* when such organisms have been identified, while continuing to employ *sea bathers' eruption* for cases in which no specified organism has been implicated.

In western Africa, the Orient, and the West Indies, schistosomal infestation poses a major health problem.

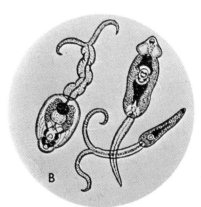

Fig. 6-1. *CERCARIAE OF SCHISTO-SOMES.* These are the immature larval form of parasitic flatworms believed to be associated with sea bathers' eruption.
Courtesy of Wiley M. Sams, M.D.

Ecologic Cycle

Cercarial dermatitis results when man becomes an unwitting interloper in a rather complex ecologic cycle. The adults of the dermatitis-producing schistosomes are blood parasites of birds or mammals. The typical cycle begins with the hatching of the schistosome eggs which are present in the droppings of infested animals.[2] Appropriate species of snails become infested upon contact with the miracidia hatched from the eggs, and the snails then serve as an intermediate host.

After a proper incubation period in the snail, hundreds of fork-tailed cercariae are released into the water and a specific warm-blooded host is found.[3] The parasites then mature in the vascular system of their host.[2] This ecologic chain is completed when the adult worms produce eggs.

Worldwide schistosome cercarial dermatitis is due to the larval form of hookworm in which snails are intermediate hosts.

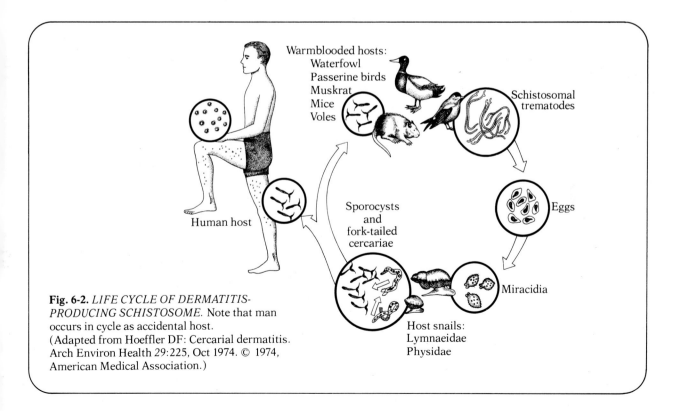

Fig. 6-2. *LIFE CYCLE OF DERMATITIS-PRODUCING SCHISTOSOME.* Note that man occurs in cycle as accidental host.
(Adapted from Hoeffler DF: Cercarial dermatitis. Arch Environ Health 29:225, Oct 1974. © 1974, American Medical Association.)

Thus, the diver or swimmer who contracts schistosome cercarial dermatitis has accidentally intruded into the normal life cycle of these parasites.

Clinical Features

Schistosome cercarial dermatitis is a skin infestation caused by an immune response in man, an unnatural host. The response induces local destruction of cercariae, producing an allergic reaction to dead cercariae.[4] The cercariae are actually walled off and destroyed in the epithelial layers of the skin. Although penetration of cercariae may take place in the water, it usually occurs as the film of water evaporates on the skin.[4]

Wood, Srolovitz, and Schetman describe the histopathology as follows: "The cercariae are apparently unable to penetrate beyond the papillary dermis; histological examination of infested tissue shows intraepithelial burrows and abscesses surrounded by and filled with eosinophils, polymorphonuclear leukocytes, and lymphocytes. Cercariae themselves are not seen in serial sections."[1]

The patient initially experiences a prickling sensation, followed by rapid development of urticarial wheals. These wheals subside in about half an hour, leaving minute macules. Severe itching and edema occur after some hours. Transformation of macules into papules—and occasionally pustules—reaches maximum intensity in two to three days. The papular and sometimes hemorrhagic rash heals in one to two weeks but may be complicated by excoriated lesions. Secondary infection with the formation of purulent lesions is common.

Barnes describes cercarial dermatitis as "essentially a sensitization phenomenon."[4] He notes that local skin lesions produced by the schistosomes of man are slight, but with continuous reinfestation, sensitized persons may show a definite dermatitis. Repeated infestations tend to become increasingly severe.

There has been some discussion as to whether the dermatitis-producing schistosome cercariae of North America can also induce systemic infestation. Most commentators have dismissed this possibility.[1]

Schistosome cercarial dermatitis, characterized by a papulourticarial eruption, often becomes pustular in nature. Secondary infection is common.

Treatment

Brisk rubbing with a rough towel is helpful as it removes water droplets harboring the cercariae. Children should be reminded to dry themselves thoroughly since they constantly enter and leave the water and often do not dry themselves properly.

Application of rubbing alcohol or equal parts of rubbing alcohol and calamine lotion is sufficient to control itching and dermatitis in milder cases. Severe cases may require systemic corticosteroids. The presence of secondary bacterial infection is an indication for antibiotics.

As with many dermatoses acquired in the course of water activities, prevention of schistosome cercarial dermatitis is the best cure. Prophylaxis should be directed toward control of intermediate molluscan hosts and their aquatic environment. Snails may be destroyed by removal of vegetation and by molluscicides. Bathers,

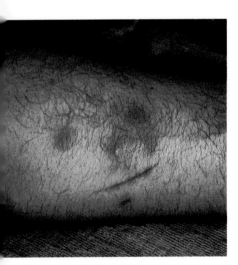

Fig. 6-3. *SCHISTOSOME DERMA-TITIS.* This eruption was caused by *Gigantobilharzia cercariae.* The papules appeared 24 hours after penetration of the schistosome. Courtesy of Harvey D. Blankespoor

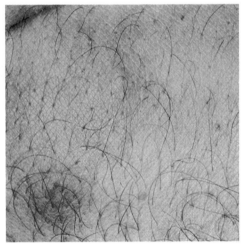

Fig. 6-4. *SCHISTOSOME DERMA-TITIS.* Papules caused by *Giganto-bilharzia* 24 hours post penetration shown at a higher magnification than seen in the previous photograph. Courtesy of Harvey D. Blankespoor

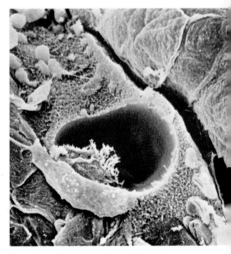

Fig. 6-5. *AVIAN SCHISTOSOME PENETRATION.* A three-dimensional view of an opening in the skin left by a cercaria of *Gigantobilharzia huronesis* following penetration (photo obtained by microscopic scanning). Courtesy of Harvey D. Blankespoor

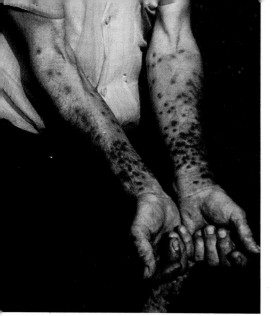

Fig. 6-6. *CERCARIAL DERMATITIS.* The eruption appeared on the arms of a patient exposed to avian schistosome cercariae while sitting on a dock jutting out over a lake. Courtesy of Harvey D. Blankespoor

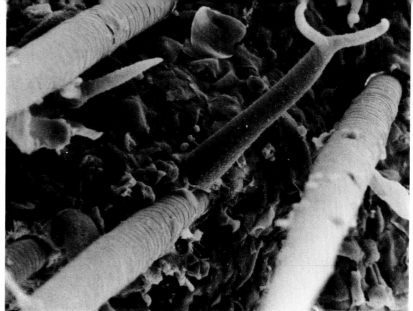

Fig. 6-7. *CERCARIA OF SCHISTOSOME* shown penetrating skin of a 10-day-old mouse. Other tubular structures are hairs. Courtesy of Harvey D. Blankespoor

So-called "sea-bathers' eruption," a dermatitis of unknown origin, resembles schistosome cercarial eruptions and seaweed dermatitis. It usually occurs on covered parts of the body.

and especially those whose occupation involves contact with infested waters, may be protected by allowing a 20% solution of copper sulfate to evaporate on the skin prior to entering such waters.

Sea Bathers' Eruption

As previously indicated, sea bathers' eruption is properly used to describe a dermatitis resulting from contact with sea water, clinically similar to cercarial dermatitis, but not traceable to cercarial penetration. Table 6-1, listing the differences between swimmers' itch and sea bathers' eruption, is presented as an aid to differential diagnosis. Sea bathers' eruption must also be distinguished from algae dermatitis, since both are mainly confined to areas covered by the bathing costume. It would appear that sea bathers' eruption is caused by some organism that can be brushed off before it penetrates the skin.

The acute dermatitis begins a short time after bathing in the sea. Erythematous macules, papules, or wheals are observed within a few hours after exposure. These lesions are localized on covered parts such as the abdomen, buttocks, and thighs, and on the breasts of female patients. Accompanying symptoms may include chills, a low-grade 24-hour temperature, a burning sensation and pruritus.

Some patients suffer repeatedly following seawater bathing, while

Table 6-1

Contrast Between Swimmers' Itch and Sea Bathers' Eruption*

Factor	Swimmers' Itch	Sea Bathers' Eruption
Type of water	Fresh	Salt
Part of body involved	Uncovered	Covered
Locale	Northern U.S., Canada	Florida, Cuba
Cause	Schistosome (?)	Unknown

*Fisher AA: Aquatic contact dermatitis, in Fisher AA: *Contact Dermatitis*, ed 2. Phila-delphia, Lea & Febiger, 1973, p 344.

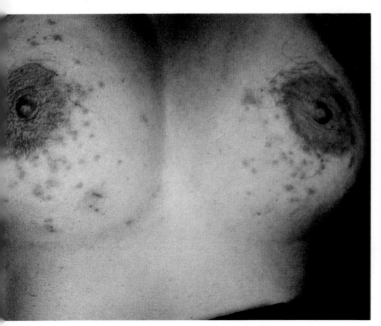

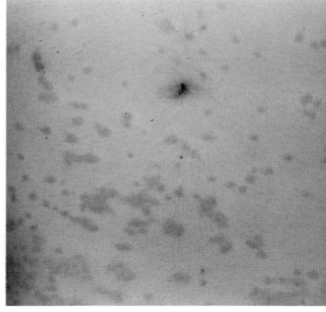

Fig. 6-8. *SEA BATHERS' ERUPTION.* The dermatitis begins a short time after bathing in the sea. Erythematous macules, papules, or wheals are observed within a few hours after exposure. The associated pruritus is at times severe, but it subsides in a few days without giving rise to further difficulty.

Fig. 6-9. *SEA BATHERS' ERUPTION.* In this close-up view of the abdomen, it can be seen that the eruption occurs predominantly on those parts of the body covered by the bathing suit (in this case, a one-piece suit).
Courtesy of Wiley M. Sams, M.D.

other swimmers in the same area remain unaffected—suggesting that individual susceptibility or sensitization may be operative. Other than avoiding swimming in infested waters, the only practical method of prophylaxis consists of wiping the skin dry on emerging from the water.

The disorder is usually self-limiting, rarely persisting for more than seven to ten days. Therapy is palliative, consisting of calamine lotion with 1% menthol. Parenteral antihistamines usually control the eruption and itching. Rarely, systemic corticosteroids may be required.

Leeches

Leeches have played a Jekyll and Hyde role in the existence of man. In its Jekyll guise, the medicinal leech was used routinely for blood-letting from ancient times until the last century. In many areas of the world, it is still a time-honored therapy.

In its Hyde aspect, the leech has been implicated in a number of disastrous historical events. Tennent[6] describes how land leeches routed an entire battalion of English soldiers from their wooded encampment in Ceylon. Harmer and Shipley[7] report on a genus of freshwater leeches, *Limnatis,* which harrassed Napoleon's soldiers in the Nile region.

Leeches are classified in the phylum Annelida (segmented worms) in which they constitute the class Hirudinea. They can be further categorized under marine, freshwater, and terrestrial types. Marine leeches have a saltwater habitat and feed on fishes. Freshwater leeches—still used as therapeutic agents in certain regions—are present in lakes, ponds, and creeks. Terrestrial leeches are especially common in tropical rain forests.

Leeches attach themselves to the skin, feed until engorged, then fall off to the ground. At the site of attachment, the leech introduces an anticoagulant, hirudin, as well as antigenic substances that have not been specifically identified. The leech draws out blood in considerable excess of its maximum needs.

The wound bleeds freely and heals slowly in unsensitized individuals, even when not infected by pyogenic organisms. If sensitization has developed, reaction to the bite may be urticarial, bullous, or necrotic. Heldt reports that the bite of the leech can cause serious

Marine, freshwater and terrestrial leeches introduce hirudin, an anticoagulant, which can act as a sensitizer and produce allergic reactions. Application of alcohol facilitates removal and prevents jaws of leeches from remaining in the wound.

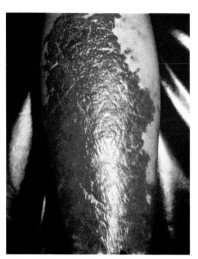

Fig. 6-10. *HEMORRHAGIC REACTION TO LEECHES.* When a leech attaches itself to the skin, it introduces an anticoagulant, hirudin, as well as antigenic substances that have not been specifically identified. The wound bleeds freely and heals slowly in unsensitized individuals.

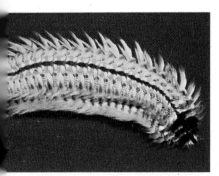

Fig. 6-11. *BRISTLE WORM* equipped with tufts of silky chitinous bristles arranged in rows around its body. When the worm is touched or stimulated in some other fashion, the bristles are raised in defense, and the body of the worm contracts simultaneously.
Courtesy of the Miami Seaquarium

allergic reactions, including anaphylaxis.[8]

Individuals walking through streams or marshes are the usual victims of leech bites; in areas where leeches are still employed medicinally, allergic reactions may complicate treatment.

Removal of leeches may be facilitated by application of a few drops of brine, alcohol or strong vinegar, or a match flame applied near the site of attachment. These measures force the leech to release its hold. Leeches should never be pulled off the skin, lest the jaws remain in the wounds and induce phagedenic ulcers. Bleeding from the bites may be staunched with a styptic pencil. Infection can be prevented by bathing the wounds for several days with mild antiseptic lotions, such as boric acid solution or calamine lotion with 25% alcohol.

Marine Annelid Dermatitis

A number of marine organisms can produce an irritant dermatitis or wound either by contact with their bristles or by the bite from their jaws.

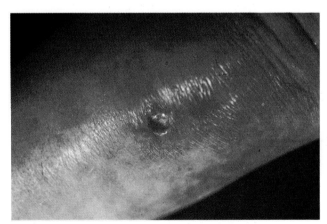

Fig. 6-12. *NECROTIC REACTION TO BRISTLE WORM.* Occasionally necrotic lesions follow a bristle worm "sting."

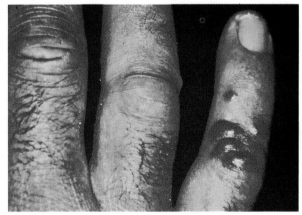

Fig. 6-13. *BRISTLE WORM INJURY.* Contact with the bristle worm produced a burning sensation accompanied by moderate edema and a papular eruption. Itching, pain and paresthesia are frequent symptoms.
Courtesy of William Orris, M.D.

Bristle Worm Dermatitis

Certain sea worms belonging to the family Amphinomidae are equipped with tufts of silky chitinous bristles arranged in rows around their bodies. When these worms are touched or stimulated in some other fashion, the bristles are raised in defense, and the body of the worm contracts simultaneously. Thus, an almost continuous defensive armor of bristles is presented to those who disturb the worm.

These bristles detach easily, penetrating the skin in much the same way as the spines of the prickly pear cactus. The spines are as difficult to remove as cactus spines; each spine has to be removed individually.

The common bristle worm of the lower east coast of Florida and the Florida Keys is *Hermodice carunculata* Kinberg. Commonly attaining a length of a foot or more and nearly an inch wide, this species is generally found on coral, rock slabs, sponges, and in porous rock. The worm itself is green with reddish markings along the sides, and the white bristles are tipped with dull red. Although the bristle-tufts appear small when the worm is not in a fighting mood, these white tufts "blossom" impressively when *H. carunculata* is disturbed.

Amphinema brasiliensis resembles *H. carunculata* except that the gills are red; their bristle stings are similar.

In contrast to *Hermodice*—which is a sea bottom worm—*Chloeia euglochis* Ehlers is a freely swimming bristle worm often found near the water surface, swimming by means of short, wave-like undulations. There are instances of *Chloeia* being caught on a hook as they attempt to settle on the bait.[9]

In various parts of the world, the following worms produce a bristle-worm dermatitis:

Chloeia flava (Pallas)	Malayan coast
Chloeia viridis (Schmarda)	West Indies, Gulf of California, Mexico south to Panama
Euythoe complanata (Pallas)	Australia and the tropical seas
Hermodice carunculata (Pallas)	tropical eastern America and eastern Gulf of Mexico.

Map 6-1.
Primary Geographic Distribution of Some Dermatitis-Producing Bristle Worms

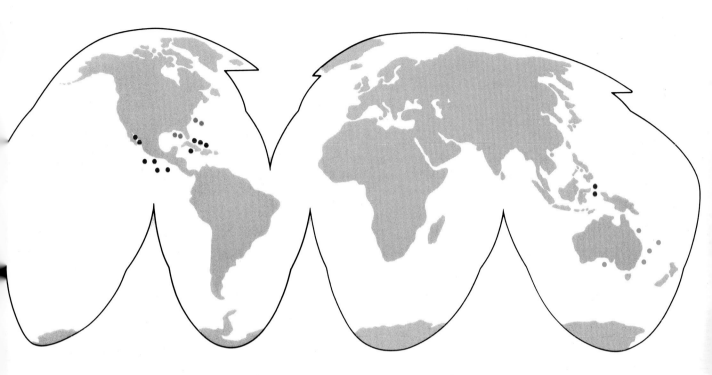

● *Chloeia flava*
● *Chloeia viridis*
● *Euythoe complanata*
● *Hermodice carunculata*

69

Contact with a bristle worm produces a burning sensation accompanied by moderate edema, a papular eruption, and occasionally necrotic lesions. Itching, pain and paresthesia are frequent symptoms.

In treating worm "stings," the bristles must be carefully removed with forceps. Scraping is usually ineffective, as the bristles tend to break off and remain embedded in the skin. However, an effective method of removing bristles is to cover them with adhesive tape. When the tape is pulled off, the attached bristles are usually removed with it. Following removal, application of diluted ammonia water or alcohol can be soothing. In an emergency situation, rubbing the affected area may have an immediate palliative effect.

Worm Bites

Certain segmented worms bite with chitinous jaws, producing a stinging pain. Edema and itching may follow. The application of cold compresses or alcohol is soothing. Handling of any sea worms should be avoided unless gloves are worn.

Contact with the bristle worm produces papular edematous lesions. Removal of bristles is facilitated with adhesive tape. Alcohol should be applied.

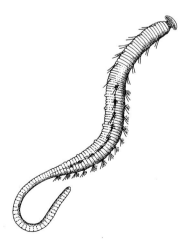

Chapter VI — References:

1. Wood MG, Srolovitz H, Schetman D: Schistosomiasis: Paraplegia and ectopic skin lesions as admission symptoms. *Arch Derm 112*:690, May 1976.
2. Chu GWT: Pacific area distribution of freshwater and marine cercarial dermatitis. *Pacific Sci 12*:299, 1958.
3. Hoeffler DF: Cercarial dermatitis. *Arch Environ Health 29*:225, Oct. 1974.
4. Barnes, RD: Invertebrate Zoology. Clinical Parasitology. Appleton Century Crofts, W. B. Saunders Co., Philadelphia, 1958, p. 632.
5. Sams WM: Seabathers' eruption. *Arch Derm Syph 60*:227, 1949.
6. Tennent JE: Ceylon, an account of the island, physical, historical, and topographical, with notes on its natural history, antiquities, and productions. London, Longman, Green, Longman & Roberts, 1859, vol 1, p 305.
7. Harmer SF, Shipley AE: Cambridge Natural History. London, Macmillan, 1896, vol 2, pp 406-408.
8. Heldt TJ: Allergy to leeches. *Henry Ford Hosp Med Bull 9*:498, 1961.
9. Phillips C, and Brady WH: Sea pests, poisonous or harmful sea life of Florida and the West Indies. Univ. Miami Press, Miami, 1953, p 247.

Injuries and Eruptions Caused by Venomous Fish Spines and Fish Skin

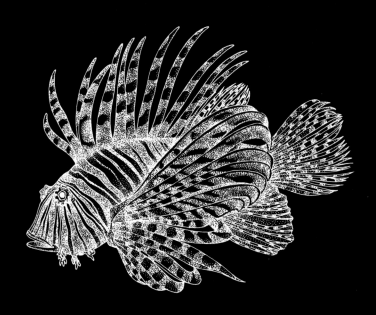

Lionfish *Pterois volitans*

Injuries and Eruptions Caused by Venomous Fish Spines and Fish Skin

Many beach-goers, including children, enjoy themselves by indulging in recreational activities other than swimming. Chief among these are wading and strolling along the beach.

While engaging in these apparently harmless pastimes, it is not unusual for the wader or beach stroller to happen upon a round or diamond-shaped creature with a whip-like tail. The unwary person may kick at the creature or accidentally step on it—acts that may be regretted. The person has struck a stingray, a sea animal whose defensive weaponry includes venomous spines capable of inducing severe skin eruptions and systemic reactions that can be fatal.

The stingray is only one of many species of fish that can inflict painful and dangerous lacerations by means of dorsal or caudal spines equipped with complex venom glands. In warm waters, scorpion fish, catfish, rabbitfish, stargazers, and toadfish (in addition to the stingray) are among the most common causes of poison spine dermatitis.

In cold waters, the weever, the spiny dogfish, the Norway haddock, and several species of stingray can inflict serious wounds.

General Clinical Features*

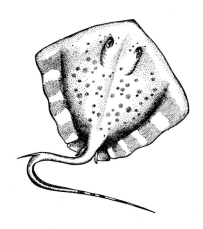

Patients who sustain punctures and lacerations from fish spines may experience intense pain for several hours. Edema and erythema in the area of the penetrated skin may simulate bacterial cellulitis. These wounds, notoriously slow in healing, often become infected. Venomous spines of several species produce rapid and severe systemic symptoms. Shock, vomiting, abdominal pain, profuse sweating, and tachycardia may be followed by muscular paralysis and death.

General Treatment †

The chemical and pharmacologic nature of fish spine venom has not been adequately elucidated. It does appear, however, that the venom is heat–labile. As a general rule, therefore, wounds from

---

*Clinical features of fish spine venom eruptions associated with specific species are described in the appropriate subsection.
†Treatment of specific fish envenomizations is described further on.

First aid treatment of puncture wounds produced by venomous fish spines consists of soaking the injured area in water as hot as can be tolerated.

poison fish spines should be treated with heat. Keep involved extremities at rest, and treat infected wounds with antibiotics.

Stingray Envenomization

Depicted as "demons of the sea," "denizens of the deep," or "devil fishes," stingrays are elasmobranchs which have been recognized as venomous since ancient times.[1] They were known to Aristotle and Pliny; Dioscorides (circa 100 B.C.) gave the first detailed description of convulsions and death due to stingray envenomization.[2] Eleven species of stingrays have been identified on the coasts of the United States: seven in the Atlantic Ocean and four in the Pacific Ocean.

These flat, smooth sea creatures have a characteristic round, kite, or diamond shape and a long whip-like tail. They range in size from a diameter of several inches to a breadth of 4 to 5 feet. *Dasyatis sabina*, especially abundant in Tampa Bay, reaches a maximum breadth of about a foot.[3] Other species may attain a length of over 14 feet. Most people afflicted with stingray wounds acquire them via contact with the smaller species which frequent shallow waters around rocky areas and burrow themselves in the sand.[4]

Stingrays are mainly scavengers, feeding on small crustaceans and fish scraps. They glide slowly about with alternate wing-like motions of their pectoral fins. When they come to rest with a sud-

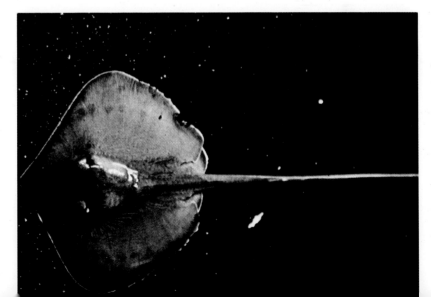

Fig. 7-1. *ATLANTIC STINGRAY.* Freshwater stingrays of this type are found in the great Atlantic rivers of tropical and temperate South America and Equatorial Africa. These smooth sea creatures have a characteristic round, kite, or diamond shape and a long whip-like tail. Courtesy of the Miami Seaquarium

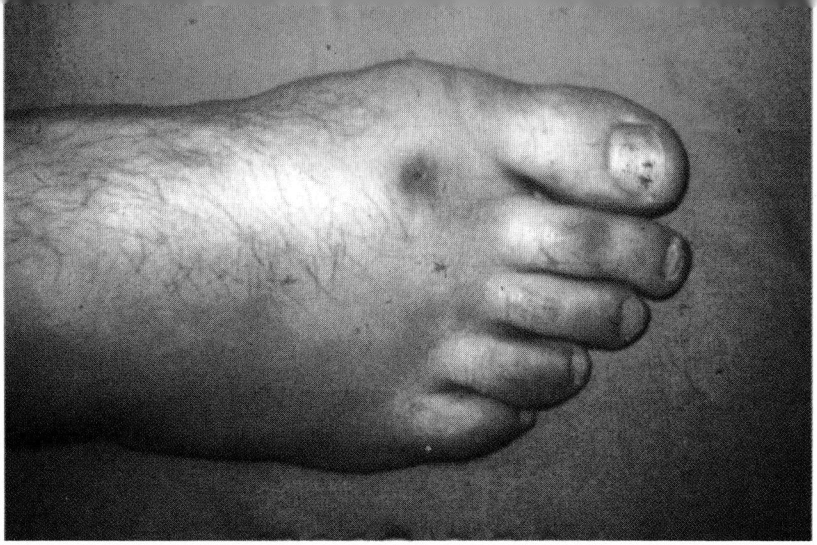

Fig. 7-2. *STINGRAY WOUND.* Discoloration of the skin is generally not pronounced immediately following injury, but within two hours erythema and violaceous color appear around the edges of the wound. This may extend several centimeters. Courtesy of Bruce W. Halstead, M.D. and Maurice B. Strauss, M.D.

The venomous spines of the stingray are located in the animal's tail which lashes forcefully in response to danger.

den quick movement of the fins, they stir up a cloud of sand which covers their entire body except for their eyes. Stingrays are not aggressive. When startled, the ray will usually hasten away at great speed, leaving behind a muddy wake. But their habit of lying motionless in shallow water—virtually covered with sand—makes them easily stepped on by the unwary bather or wader.

Venom Apparatus

The "sting" of the stingray is a bilaterally serrated, dentinal caudal spine located on the dorsum of the animal's tail. Within this dentinal structure are venomous canals containing loose, reticular tissues and small, thin-walled blood vessels. A thin layer of compact matrix is seen at the surface of the spine.[1] The spine is encased in an integumentary sheath and the venom is contained within the ventrolateral grooves.

When accidentally stepped on, pressure of the foot on the dorsum of the fish provokes it to thrust its tail upward and forward, driving its sting into the victim's foot or leg. When the sting enters the flesh, the integumentary sheath is ruptured, releasing the venom into the victim's tissues. As the spine is withdrawn, the integumentary sheath may be torn free and remain embedded in the wound.

Symptomatology

Stingray wounds may be large and severely lacerated. Russell[1] reports that a sting no wider than 5 mm may produce a wound approximately 3 cm long, and larger stings may produce wounds as long as 7 inches.

Patients stung by stingrays (usually in the foot or leg) describe the experience as similar to having received a sharp painful stab. The stinging is followed by the immediate onset of intense pain. The pain can be quite excruciating, increasing in severity during the first 90 minutes following contact. The pain appears to be out of proportion to that which might be produced by nonvenomous fish or by stepping on a broken bottle or bivalve.

Examination generally reveals a freely bleeding puncture or laceration, often contaminated with parts of the stingray's integumentary sheath. Discoloration is generally not pronounced immediately following the injury, but within two hours discoloration around the edges may extend several centimeters from the wound. If left untreated, necrosis of this area is fairly common. Edema is a frequent finding and may persist for several weeks in untreated patients.

Although symptoms and signs of envenomization are usually localized to the injured area, a number of systemic symptoms can occur. These range from syncope, weakness, nausea, and anxiety, to generalized cramps, fasciculations in the muscles of the affected extremity, inguinal or axillary pain, and respiratory distress. Arrhythmias, paresthesia, and convulsions may also occur.[1]

Treatment

The wound should be debrided, and heat should be applied immediately—preferably by immersion in hot water or by means of hot wet compresses. High temperatures may be attained if the extremity is first immersed in comfortably hot water; then hotter water can be added as acclimatization takes place.

Relief from pain is usually immediate. Continue hot soaking for at least 30 minutes, and repeat if the pain returns. Occasionally, several heat treatments may prove necessary to neutralize all the venom present.

In severe envenomization, a tourniquet induces slow venous return and may be lifesaving. Use elastic material applied just tight enough to allow insertion of the index finger under the tourniquet and loosen for 90 seconds every 10 minutes.

Treatment for shock may be necessary, and respiratory stimu-

Stingray injuries produce intense localized pain which may be followed by necrosis and persistent edema in the untreated patient.

lants may have to be administered.

Patients should be advised to exercise considerable care when wading in shallow waters known to be inhabited by stingrays.

Freshwater Rays

Freshwater stingrays are found in the great Atlantic rivers of tropical and temperate South America and Equatorial Africa and in the Mekong River of Laos.[5] In all of these regions, the sting of the freshwater rays are greatly feared. Stingrays are widely distributed in streams of the Amazon River and Rio de la Plata (Plate River), and numerous stories and superstitions attest to the fear inspired by this creature in pioneers and Indians.[6] The subject of freshwater stingray envenomization has been intensively studied only in recent years. General clinical features and treatment measures appear to be similar to those associated with envenomization caused by saltwater species.

Scorpion Fish Envenomization

Scorpion fishes are the most venomous of all fish. The spine venom found in several species which inhabit tropical seas—especially the venom of the notorious stonefish, *Synanceja*—has been compared to cobra venom in its neurotoxicity. The stonefish has been justifiably described as the most dangerous of all stinging fishes.

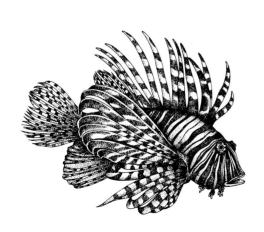

Members of the family Scorpaenidae, scorpion fishes have been classified into 350 separate species, including the lionfish, zebrafish, bullrout, and waspfish. Widely distributed throughout all tropical and most temperate seas, the greatest number of species are found in the tropical Indo-Pacific. Some scorpion fishes closely resemble sea bass, while others are exquisitely modified to mimic patches of seaweed in shape and color. The most dangerous are remarkably camouflaged to resemble algae-covered rocks or to blend in with the small coral masses among which they live.[3]

Although the spine venom of local species of scorpion fishes is less toxic than that of Indo-Pacific species, it should be remembered that they are nonetheless highly venomous and have the potential to cause severe dermatologic and systemic effects. Scorpion fishes are common about the Florida Keys, Caribbean, Gulf of Mexico, and Southern California; the California species is often

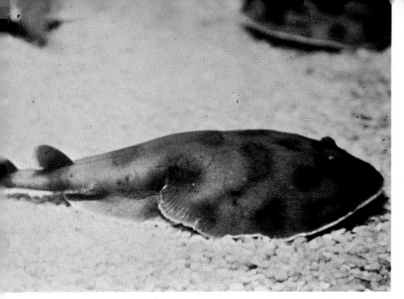

Fig. 7-3. *TORPEDO RAY,* one of eleven species of saltwater stingrays identified on the coasts of the U.S.
Courtesy of the Miami Seaquarium

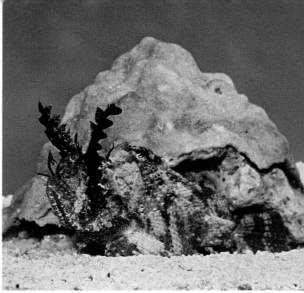

Fig. 7-4. *LIONFISH.* This member of the scorpion fish family is found in the Atlantic. The most dangerous of the Scorpaenidae are remarkably camouflaged to resemble alga-covered rocks or to blend in with the small coral masses among which they live.
Courtesy of the Miami Seaquarium

The poison spines of scorpion fish produce a wound which should be treated like snakebite, and for which an antivenin is available.

called "sculpin."

The venom of scorpion fishes is contained within the tissues which envelop certain of the dorsal, pelvic, and anal fin spines. The number of venomous spines varies with the species, as does the structure of the venom gland or venom-containing tissues. Envenomization occurs from mechanical pressure on the spine which tears the integumentary sheath and allows the venom to escape into the wound.[7]

Because of their protective coloring and their habit of lying motionless on the rocky bottoms or burying themselves in the sand, scorpion fishes are easily stepped on. When this occurs, the spine sheaths are depressed and the poison glands are stimulated into releasing their contents; the stinging action is virtually automatic.

Intense pain, localized swelling, discoloration, and paresthesia around the wound are common reactions. Systemic symptoms and signs may include lymphadenitis, nausea, vomiting, weakness, pallor, and syncope. Untreated patients may suffer respiratory distress, shock, and coma.

First aid treatment for scorpion fish stings is similar to that employed in cases of snakebite. The wound should be opened with a knife or lancet and the surrounding area squeezed or sucked to remove as much poison as possible. Sucking with the lips will not have harmful effects, since any poison which may be swallowed is quickly neutralized by stomach acids. If bleeding is not too profuse, it can be allowed to continue for a minute or two. However, prolonged bleeding should be stopped by placing a tourniquet at the nearest joint adjacent to the wound.

Immersion of the limb in hot water may bring symptomatic relief when other measures have failed.

The Commonwealth Laboratories of Parkville, Victoria, Australia, have made available an antivenin for the treatment of stonefish spine poisoning.

Catfish Envenomization

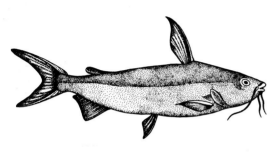

The ability of catfish to inflict extremely painful wounds with their pectoral and dorsal spines has been well established over a period of many decades. While most of the documented stings have resulted from contact with saltwater species, freshwater catfish—quite abundant in the rivers and streams of North America—can also administer a painful and very distressing sting to humans.[8]

The common sea catfish, *Galeichthys felis*, has four barbels on its chin. Its body is smooth and scaleless, dark silvery gray above and white beneath, and it spans a length of about a foot. A shore fish, it prefers the muddy areas around docks and boat-slips. The ability of catfishes to eat and digest virtually any food they can swallow is almost legendary.

Although the North American marine species are rarely eaten, our freshwater catfishes are commonly included in the diets of many Americans. Freshwater catfishes of North America include the brown bullhead, the Carolina mudtom, the channel catfish, the blue catfish, and the white catfish. All are primarily bottom feeders, with the same lack of discrimination in diet as their saltwater cousins.

The venom apparatus of the saltwater catfish includes dorsal and pectoral stings and the axillary venom glands. Dorsal and pectoral stings are comprised of modified or coalescent soft rays which have become ossified. In most catfishes, these spines are so constructed that they can be locked in the extended position at the will of the fish. Thus, the creature is equipped with a formidable and efficient defensive weapon.[9]

The victim of catfish envenomization experiences an instanta-

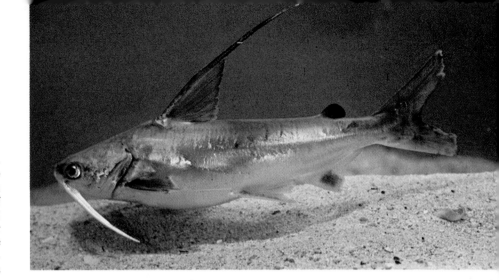

Fig. 7-5. *GAFF-TOPSAIL CATFISH*. The ability of catfish to inflict extremely painful wounds with their pectoral and dorsal spines has been well established over a period of many decades. Dorsal and pectoral spines are comprised of modified or coalescent soft rays which have become ossified.
Courtesy of the Miami Seaquarium

Fig. 7-6. *STONEFISH*, usually measuring less than one foot in length and weighing about two pounds, is one of the most dangerous stinging fish. Its venom has been compared to cobra venom in neurotoxicity.

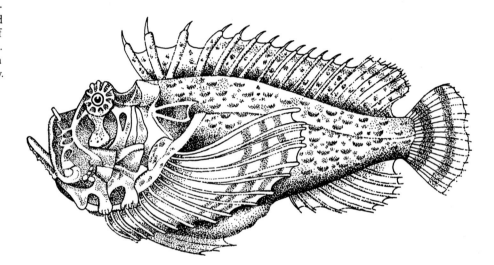

Fig. 7-7. *SCULPIN FISH* may occasionally produce a punctate dermatitis if handled.

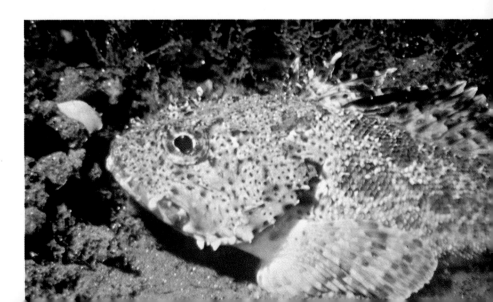

neous stinging, throbbing, or scalding sensation which may be localized or which may radiate up the affected limb. Severity of symptoms varies with the species of catfish and the amount of venom received. Discomfort produced by the less toxic species generally subsides within 30 minutes or less, whereas the more potent tropical species may produce a violent pain lasting 48 hours or more.

Immediately after the patient is stung, the area surrounding the wound becomes ischemic. The pallor is followed by a cyanotic appearance, then by redness and swelling. Patients with extreme wounds may develop a massive edema involving an entire limb, accompanied by lymphadenopathy, numbness, and localized gangrene.

Primary shock may be manifested by such symptoms as faintness, rapid weak pulse, low blood pressure, and respiratory distress.

The sting of North American catfishes is generally mild in nature, with symptoms subsiding within several hours. Although sequelae are rare, necrosis of the involved tissues has been observed with severe envenomization. Improper wound care may result in secondary bacterial infection.[10]

Therapy is symptomatic. The treatment of choice is immersion in hot water,[11] although potent analgesia may be necessary in severe cases.[8] Infections are treated with appropriate antibiotics.

Patten[11] reports that most catfishermen in the Gulf of Mexico region carry a thermos of hot water in their boat as the specific remedy to apply if they are stung.

Fish Skin Dermatitis

The skins of several fish species contain substances that are dermatologically toxic.

Scombroid Dermatitis

Scombroid dermatitis is due to a primary irritant found in the skin and flesh of scombroid fish, which include tuna, skipjack, and bonito. This dermatitis appears in workers handling scombroid fishes without wearing gloves. The irritant appears to be more concentrated in spoiled than in fresh fish.

Scombroid dermatitis and red feed dermatitis are irritant occupational hazards of fishermen who handle scombroid fish or certain mackerel without gloves.

The irritant dermatitis of the hands is treated with the application of corticosteroid cream. In the presence of fissures and denuded, excoriated or infected skin, an erythromycin ointment should also be applied.

Red Feed Dermatitis

Red feed is a reddish orange crustacean (*Calanus* species) eaten by mackerel from June to September. Ingested red feed accelerates the proteolytic breakdown of the gastric wall of the fish, releasing the gastric juices. Handling of fish which have eaten red feed results in edema, erythema, and superficial ulcerations of the skin of the hands.

The dermatitis can be counteracted by application of cold compresses and erythromycin ointment.

Map 7-1.
Primary Geographic Distribution of Stingrays.

Note that stingrays are largely concentrated in the warmer latitudes.
(Adapted from Halstead BW: Poisonous and Venomous Marine Animals of the World. Vol 3. Washington, DC, US Government Printing Office, 1965, p 146.)

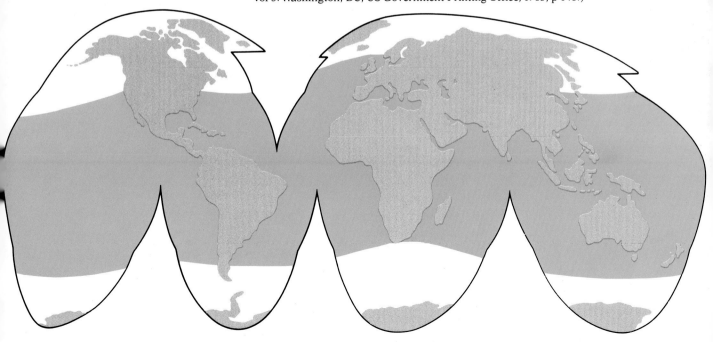

Map 7-2.
Primary Geographic Distribution of Venomous Scorpion Fish.

Scorpion fish family

Stonefish Synanceja

(Adapted from Halstead BW: Poisonous and Venomous Marine Animals of the World. Vol 3. Washington, DC, US Government Printing Office, 1965, p 428.)

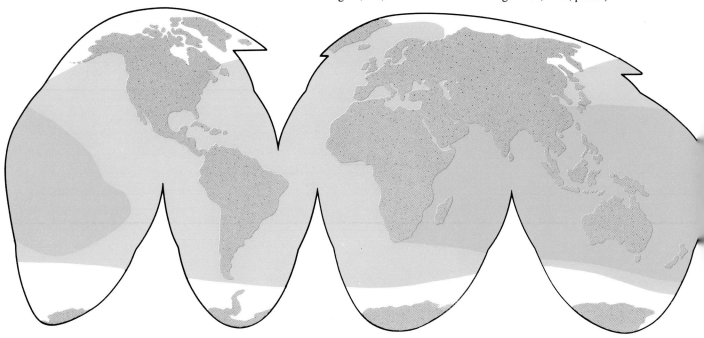

Chapter VII—References:

1. Russell FE: The stingray: National history, venom apparatus, chemistry and toxicology, and clinical problem, in Poisonous Marine Animals. Neptune, NJ, T.F.H. Publications, Inc, 1971.

2. Gudger EW: Is the stingray's sting poisonous? A historical résumé showing the development of our knowledge that it is poisonous. *Bull Hist 14*:467, 1943.

3. Phillips C, and Brady WH: Sea Pests, Poisonous or Harmful Sea Life of Florida and the West Indies. Miami, Univ Miami Press, 1953.

4. Mullanney PJ: Treatment of stingray wounds. *Clin Toxicol 3*:613, Dec 1970.

5. Castex MN: Freshwater venomous rays, in Russell FE, Saunders PR (eds): Animal Toxins: International Symposium on Animal Toxins. New York, Pergamon Press, 1967, p 167.

6. Rodrigues RJ: Pharmacology of South American freshwater stingray venom *(Potamotrygon Motoro). Trans NY Acad Sci 34*:677, 1972.

7. Schaeffer RC, Jr, Carlson RW, Russell FE: Some chemical properties of the venom of the scorpionfish *Scorpaena Guttata. Toxicon 9*:69, 1971.

8. Scoggin CH: Catfish stings. *JAMA 231*:176, Jan 13, 1975.

9. Halstead BW, Kuninobu LS, Hebard HG: Catfish stings and the venom apparatus of the Mexican catfish, *Galeichthys Felis* (Linnaeus). *Trans Am Microscopical Soc 72*:297, Oct 1953.

10. Wintrobe MM, Thorne GW, Adams RD, *et al.*: Harrison's Principles of Internal Medicine, ed 7. New York, McGraw-Hill Book Co, 1974.

11. Patten BM: More on catfish stings (letter). *JAMA 232*:248, April 21, 1975.

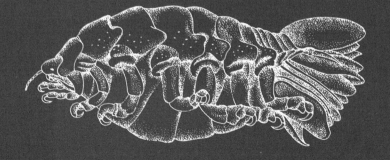

Sea louse *Lironeca puhi*

Dermatitis Caused by Other Macroscopic Organisms

The bite of the sea louse typically produces hemorrhagic punctate wounds.

Sea Louse Dermatitis

While water skiers, skin divers, and swimmers who frequent the waters of the Southern California coast have long been acquainted with the sharp bite of "sea lice," sea louse dermatitis (cymothoidism) has only recently found its way into the medical literature.[1]

Sea lice are actually small marine crustaceans of the order Isopoda, suborder Cymothoidea. These active and free swimming crustaceans generally inhabit the shoal waters of tropical and temperate estuarial shore lines.[2]

Frequently burying themselves in the sandy bottom below the water level, cymothoids will readily prey on any organism which intrudes on their immediate domain.[3] Although they usually feed upon higher marine animals, "sea lice" will also, as suggested, attack humans.

Cymothoids are equipped with a powerful biting apparatus which can quickly attach itself to fish or human extremities. The bite is rapid and sharp, causing punctate hemorrhagic wounds at the site.[1]

The injured area should be cleansed with hydrogen peroxide, and an antibiotic ointment should be applied to the hemmorhagic crusts which usually form.

Prototheosis

Prototheosis is a cutaneous or disseminated infection caused by *Prototheca*, an achloric mutant of the green alga, *Chlorella*.

In general, the principal importance of algae to medicine and sanitation has been related to toxicoses and the production of an offensive odor or taste in contaminated water supplies.[4] The blue-green algae often are indicators of sewage contamination of streams or lakes.[4]

Prototheca has been found in fresh and marine water and in sewage treatment systems.[5] Although several species have been decribed, only two—*P. segbwema* and *P. wickerhamii*—have been demonstrated as pathogens in man. There is some evidence indicating that achloric mutants of other genera of algae also exist and that some may have medical significance.[6]

Prototheosis has diverse clinical manifestations. It is probable that infection is initiated via entry of the organism through pre-existing openings in the skin.

The initial lesion is a small, pruritic eczematous papule. Subsequently, a patch of atrophic, dry, depigmented skin may develop. The raised borders of the lesions are well defined and papulo-nodular. Verrucose lesions that may ultimately develop somewhat resemble the "mossy foot" seen in elephantiasis.

Prototothecosis, a dermatosis caused by colorless algae, may vary from a depigmented atrophic area to verrucose lesions. Its cure requires surgical excision.

Prototothecosis has proven to be resistant to all types of local and systemic therapy, including x-radiation. There is only one treatment for the condition: complete surgical excision of the lesion prior to lymphatic dissemination of the organisms.

The condition is most likely to occur as a result of barefoot walks in swampy areas, work with aquariums, or exposure of the skin to water from contaminated water supply systems.

Creeping Eruption

Larva migrans (creeping eruption) forms superficial, serpiginous tunnels in the skin. Inhabitants of endemic areas should be cautioned against walking barefoot on the beach during rainy periods.

In man, creeping eruption is caused by larval hookworms of the species *Ancylostoma brasiliense, Uncinaria stenocephala,* and perhaps *A. caninum,* which are natural parasites of dogs and cats. Most often exposed to the larva are people who frequent the beach or work under buildings, such as plumbers. Although most instances of creeping eruption in the United States have been reported from the South, cases recently have been reported from the Northeast as well.[7]

In humans, the infective larvae penetrate the skin but are apparently unable to pierce through the dermis, possibly because of a lack of the necessary enzymes.[7] Instead, the larvae migrate between the dermis and epidermis, producing tunnel-like lesions. Some larvae may remain quiescent for a time before they begin to migrate.[8] The characteristic lesion is a thread-like line, about 2-4 mm wide, reddish and slightly elevated. Acute inflammation is a frequent manifestation, accompanied by severe pruritus and pain.

Diagnosis of creeping eruption is indicated by observation of the typical serpiginous tunnels. Although the index of suspicion should be increased if the patient has been in an area where creeping eruption is prevalent, the clinician cannot automatically rule out the condition in patients who have not visited such areas.

Cryotherapy with ethyl chloride is usually effective in very mild infestations. Stubborn cases generally yield to topical application of thiabendazole.[9] In the rare instances in which topical treatment

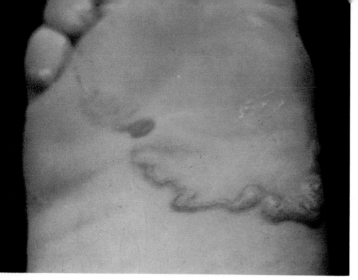

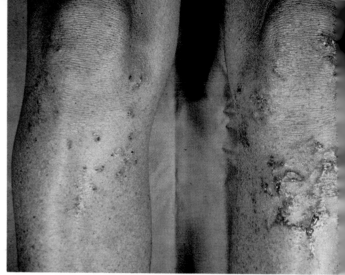

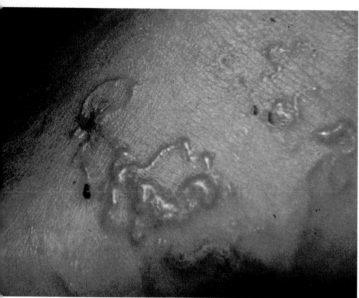

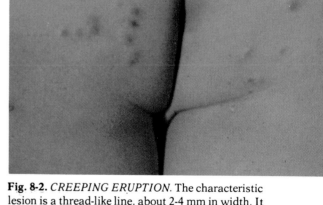

Fig. 8-1. *CREEPING ERUPTION.* This dermatosis in man is caused by larval hookworms of the species *Ancylostoma brasiliense, Uncinaria stenocephala,* and perhaps *A. caninum*—all of which are natural parasites of dogs and cats.

Fig. 8-3. *CREEPING ERUPTION.* The infective larvae apparently penetrate the skin but are unable to pierce through the dermis. Instead, the larvae migrate between the dermis and epidermis.

Fig. 8-2. *CREEPING ERUPTION.* The characteristic lesion is a thread-like line, about 2-4 mm in width. It is reddish and slightly elevated. Acute inflammation is a frequent manifestation, accompanied by severe pruritus and pain.

Fig. 8-4. *CREEPING ERUPTION.* The papular phase is shown here. Secondary infection of the skin following this phase is not uncommon. Incision and drainage of pustules or furuncles, as well as the use of topical and systemic antibiotics may be required. Courtesy of William Orris, M.D.

is ineffective, the systemic use of thiabendazole may be indicated.[10] However, such systemic administration is often accompanied by nausea and gastrointestinal side effects.

Secondary infection of skin, not uncommon in creeping eruption, may require incision and drainage of pustules or furuncles and the use of topical and systemic antibiotics.

In endemic areas, patients should be instructed in the following preventive measures:

1. Avoid sitting or lying on damp soil or sand during rainy periods; it invites infestation by the larvae.

2. Do not walk barefoot on the beach or anywhere out of doors.

3. Drape the ground with sheets of plastic, building paper, or other impervious material prior to work which involves crawling under buildings.

4. Cover sandboxes at night with a tarpaulin to prevent contamination by prowling animals.

Soapfish Dermatitis

Fishermen in the Virgin Isles and Puerto Rico are aware that keeping a soapfish in a restricted volume of sea water with other fishes often results in the death of the other fishes. Fortunately, human contact with a soapfish, *Rypticus saponaceus*, family Grammistidae, produces nothing worse than dermatitis.

The soapfish receives its name from the soapy mucus it releases when handled or otherwise disturbed. The skin irritant in this mucus is called grammistin.

Similar irritant substances have been isolated from certain species of boxfish[11] and sea bass.[12]

As with any acute irritant dermatitis, cold compresses of Burow's solution allay the burning and itching sensation produced by contact with the mucus of these fishes.

Randall[13] reports the following experience with a soapfish:

"While diving in the Florida Keys [I] became aware, in an unusual way, that something exuded from the soapfish...is very noxious. About a 9-inch (228.6 mm) adult was speared...Rather than carry the fish all the way to the boat at the surface, it was tempo-

Soapfish dermatitis is caused by grammistin—a toxin present in the soapy mucus exuded by the fish when disturbed.

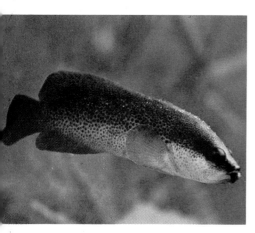

Fig. 8-5. *SOAPFISH,* so named because it produces large amounts of soapy, irritant mucus when handled or otherwise disturbed.
Courtesy of the Miami Seaquarium

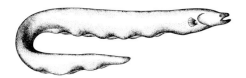

rarily stored inside [my] bathing trunks. Very soon it became apparent that a secretion from this fish was a powerful urethral irritant, and it was promptly removed from the bathing suit."

Marine Animals That Shock Electrically

Individuals who emerge from the sea in a dazed condition with no visible eruption may be suffering from electric shock produced by certain marine animals, including catfish, stargazers, electric eels, and electric rays.

These marine animals possess electricity-generating organs that can discharge 8 to 200 volts of current. The amperage is very low, and if the victim is in good health, injury is insignificant. Contact with a large marine "shocker" may result in an electric shock strong enough to knock over or temporarily disable the victim.

Recovery is usually uneventful. In severe cases, the treatment is the same as for any form of electric shock.

Chapter VIII — References:

1. Best WC, Sablan RG: Cymothoidism (sea louse dermatitis). *Arch Derm* 90:177, Aug 1964.

2. Bassler RS: Shelled invertebrates of past and present. *Smithson Sci Ser 10*:157, 1934.

3. Noble ER, Noble, GA: *Parasitology, ed. 1.* Philadelphia, Lea and Febiger, 1961, p 383.

4. Davies RR, Spencer H, Wakelin PO: A case of human protothecosis. *Trans Roy Soc Trop Med Hyg* 58:448, 1964.

5. Tindall JP, Fetter BF: Infection caused by achloric algae (protothecosis). *Arch Derm 104*:490, 1971.

6. Klintworth GK, Fetter BF, Nielsen HS Jr: Protothecosis, an algal infection: Report of a case in man. *J Med Microbiol* 1:211, 1968.

7. Stromberg BE, Christie AD: Creeping eruption and triabendazole. *Int J Derm 15*:355, 1976.

8. Stone OJ, Willis CJ: Cutaneous hookworm reservoir. *J Invest Derm* 49:237, 1967.

9. Davis CM, Israel RM: Treatment of creeping eruption with topical thiabendazole. *Arch Derm 97*:325, 1968.

10. Stone OU, Mullins JF: First use of thiabendazole in creeping eruption. *Tex Rep Biol Med 21*:422, 1963.

11. Boylan DB, Scheuer PJ: Pahutoxin: A fish poison. *Science 155*:52, Jan 6, 1967.

12. Hashimoto Y, Kamiya H: Occurrence of a toxic substance in the skin of a sea bass *Pogonoperca Punctata.* Toxicon. Great Britain, Pergamon Press, vol 7, pp 65-70.

13. Randall JE, Aida K, Hibiya T, *et al:* Grammistin, the skin toxin of soapfishes, and its significance in the classification of Grammistidae. *Publ Seto Marine Biol Lab 19*:157, 1971.

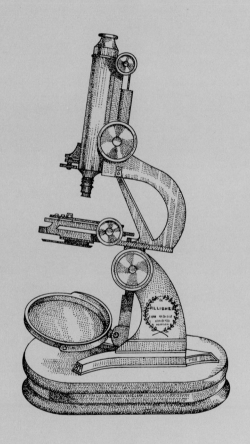

Dermatitis and Infections Caused by Marine Bacteria

Mycobacteriosis

Infections with atypical mycobacteria have been recognized for almost a century, especially in birds and cold-blooded vertebrates such as frogs, snakes and many varieties of fish. However, the pathogenicity of these organisms for man has been recognized only since the early years of this century.

In 1926, Aronson[1] described tubercles in various organs of salt-water fish found dead in the tanks of the Philadelphia Aquarium. He found acid-fast bacilli that differed from other previously known mycobacteria and named the newly identified organism *Mycobacterium marinum.*

Skin granulomas caused by *M. marinum (balnei)* were first called to the attention of physicians by Linell and Norden[2] in 1954. These authors described an epidemic of skin lesions, resembling tuberculosis verrucosa cutis, which occurred in the Swedish town of Orebro. Eighty cases were reported, 19 of which appeared about three weeks after patients had received abrasions from the wall of a swimming pool.[3]

M. marinum is an acid-fast, rod-shaped bacillus, fast growing at 24°-30°C. It is found in freshwater and seawater, and often in soil as well.[4] It is photochromogen—forming orange pigment after exposure to daylight—and has been classified in Runyon's group I.[5]

Although mycobacteriosis may result from exposure to aquariums or fish bites, the infection originates most frequently in swimming pools. Chlorinated swimming pools provide little protection, since the organism appears to be resistant to chlorine. Concentrations of 10 mg/liter of water or more are necessary for growth inhibition.[5]

M. marinum (balnei) invades the tissue through a preexisting skin lesion. The site of invasion is marked by a tender, red or bluish-red nodule, which may be as large as 6 centimeters in diameter and which occasionally becomes purulent.

New lesions may continue to appear in a pattern resembling sporotrichosis.[6] Healing may take place with scarring and pigmentation.[3]

The disease usually runs a benign course with spontaneous resolution in a few months. However, lesions may appear in the lungs, larynx, and lymph nodes and produce long-standing debility.[7]

Swimming Pool Granulomas

In the United States, individuals often develop swimming pool granulomas resulting from contact with *M. marinum (balnei)*. The most widespread epidemic of granulomatous mycobacteriosis occurred in Colorado and was described in the literature in 1963.[8] Some 290 patients, mostly teenagers, were infected from a common source—a contaminated swimming pool.

Pathogenesis

Swimming pool granulomas generally develop on the traumatized skin of the elbows, knees, and dorsal aspects of the hands and feet. The incubation period usually lasts three to four weeks, after which a small red papule can be observed. This early lesion slowly increases in size to become a hard purple nodule, sometimes ulcerating and becoming covered with a gray exudate or crust. Pain is minimal. Eventually, the lesion may become verrucose. Lymphangitis or regional lymphadenopathy is an infrequent symptom. Healing with scarring occurs after several months in most cases, although there are reports of lesions persisting for 4 to 45 years. [9,10]

Diagnosis

Frequently the offending bacillus has been isolated from crevices and grooves in the cement walls of pools in which patients had been swimming. Skin tests with a purified protein derivative (PPD) of the organism are usually positive. Cross-reactivity with the purified protein derivative of other acid-fast bacteria, particularly the tubercle bacillus, is common. Culture characteristics distinguish *M. marinum* from the tubercle bacillus.

Therapy

Treatment of swimming pool granulomas should be conservative, since most lesions heal without therapy.[11] Chemotherapy may be justified when multiple lesions are present, but it should always follow culture and sensitivity studies. Administration of ethambutol hydrochloride and cycloserine may afford symptomatic relief.

With the possible exception of ethambutol and cycloserine, the bacillus appears to be resistant to standard antituberculosis drugs. Loria[12] recently reported therapeutic success with oral administration of minocycline hydrochloride. Surgical excision may be chosen for the treatment of single, small, stubborn lesions.

Erysipelothrix Dermatitis

This dermatitis is sometimes known as erysipeloid of Rosenbach. It also has several more colorful appellations, including "speck finger" and "blubber finger." The condition is most common in fish handlers but can occur in anyone working with marine food products or aquariums. On the Atlantic Coast, erysipeloid infection frequently occurs among workers who handle crabs and live fish, and it is believed to be one of the main causes of temporary disability in such occupations.[13]

Erysipelothrix, the causative organism, is a gram-positive coccoid that later becomes a gram-positive bacillus. *E. rhusiopathiae, E. muriseptica,* and *E. erysipeloids* are either variants of the same species or the same organism. These organisms are slender rods which may be either curved or straight and which usually show elongated filaments. They are nonmotile and do not form spores or capsules.[14] Closely related bacteriologically to *Listeria*, the organism may be easily confused with streptococci or diphtheroids.

Erysipelothrix enters the skin through an opening, usually a small puncture wound on the finger. After a one- to five-day incubation period, a spreading erythema is observed, accompanied by pain and itching.[15]

Three forms of the disease have been reported: (1) a mild localized cutaneous form; (2) a severe generalized cutaneous form; and (3) a systemic form, sometimes complicated by endocarditis.

The localized form involves the fingers and hands. It begins as a sharply defined violent red area around the site or infection. Prickling, itching, and pain are frequent accompanying symptoms. Occasionally the lesion becomes purulent. Aching or burning digits may interfere with the patient's sleep.

The lesion characteristically progresses up the edge of the finger into the web and then descends the adjoining finger. It commonly spreads to the dorsum of the hand but seldom affects the palm.

Erysipeloid of Rosenbach, caused by the erysipelothrix, is an occupational hazard in workers handling crabs and live fish. Both the localized cutaneous lesions and the systemic variety usually are amenable to penicillin.

92

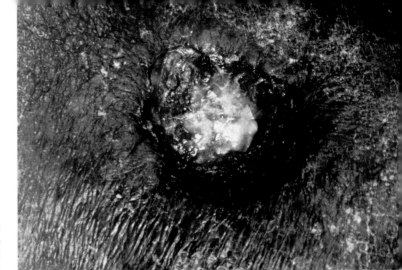

Fig. 9-1. *SWIMMING POOL GRANULOMA.*
Close-up of an ulcerated granuloma caused
by *Mycobacterium balnei.* The causative
organism is an acid-fast, rod-shaped
bacillus found in both fresh and seawater.

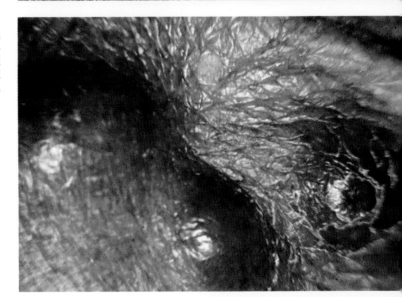

Fig. 9-2. *SWIMMING POOL GRANULOMA.*
In the typical course of this condition, a
small red papule appears after an incubation period of three to four weeks, and
slowly increases in size to become a hard
purple nodule. Just such a nodule is seen in
this photograph.
Courtesy of John Van Dyke, M.D.

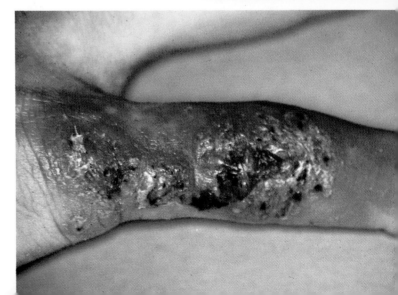

Fig. 9-3. *ULCERATED GRANULOMA OF
THE FINGER.* The swimming pool-associated condition had been present for five
years in this patient. At the time the photograph was taken, the finger had become
completely immobile.
Courtesy of Farrington Daniels, Jr., M.D.
and Sam C. Atkinson, M.D.

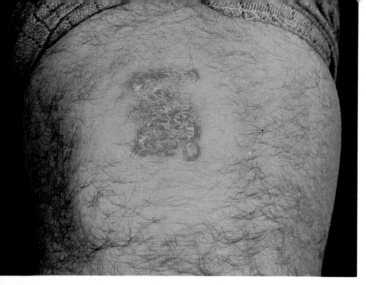

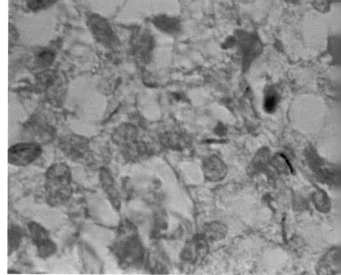

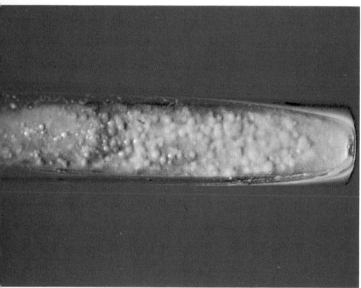

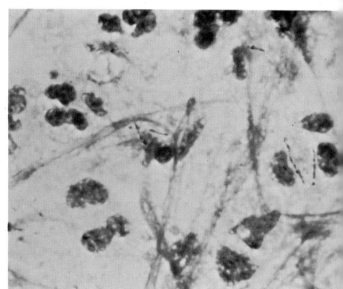

Fig. 9-4. *ATYPICAL ACID-FAST INFECTION* of the right knee. Such infections are not infrequent in the Gulf of Mexico coastal region. In making the diagnosis, granuloma annulare and lichen planus have to be differentiated. Courtesy of Philip Ronald Loria, M.D.

Fig. 9-6. *ACID-FAST BACILLI* in culture obtained from pus removed from a fish tank granuloma. Courtesy of John Van Dyke, M.D.

Fig. 9-5. *ACID-FAST BACILLI* in tissue taken from a fish tank granuloma. Courtesy of John Van Dyke, M.D.

Fig. 9-7. *ACID-FAST BACILLI* are shown in pus. The original lesion was from a fish tank granuloma. Courtesy of John Van Dyke, M.D.

Since erysipeloid is a self-limiting condition—usually running its course within one to three weeks—conservative treatment is indicated. Administration of appropriate antibiotics follows culture identification and sensitivity tests. Penicillin therapy is generally helpful. Surgery is contraindicated in most cases. Reporting on ten patients with the condition, Lamphier[16] found that duration of the disease was doubled in five patients who underwent surgery.

Pseudomonas cepacia Dermatitis

Foot lesions associated with *Pseudomonas cepacia* are variously known as jungle rot, foot rot, swamp rot or trench foot.

The organism has been isolated from lesions of the feet, hands, and groin. Invasion takes place through intact, sodden skin. Soldiers exposed to swampy, wet terrain are most frequently affected.

The lesions are characterized by maceration, hyperkeratosis, and fissuring.[17] The toe webs are often involved.

Prophylaxis consists of cleanliness and dryness. Resistance to antibiotics is characteristic of *Ps. cepacia*. Novobiocin is active *in vitro* against most strains. Chloramphenicol may be given in severe cases. All strains tested have been sensitive to readily maintained levels of trimethoprim and sulfamethoxazole combined in the ratio of 20 parts sulfamethoxazole to 1 part trimethoprim.

A severe, macerated, fissured dermatitis due to Pseudomonas cepacia occurs most often on lower extremities which have had long exposure to soggy terrain.

Chapter IX— References:

1. Aronson JD: Spontaneous tuberculosis in salt water fish. *J Infect Dis 39*:315, 1926.

2. Linell F, Norden A: *Mycobacterium balnei. Acta Tuberc Scand*, suppl 33, pp 1-84, 1954.

3. Zeligman I: *Mycobacterium marinum* granuloma. A disease acquired in the tributaries of Chesapeake Bay. *Arch Derm 106*:26, July 1972.

4. Chapman JS: The ecology of atypical mycobacteria. *Arch Environ Health 22*:41, 1971.

5. Reznikov M: Atypical mycobacteria: Their classification and aetiological significance. *Med J Aust 1*:553, 1970.

6. Dickey RF: Sporotrichoid Mycobacterium caused by *M. marinum (balnei). Arch Derm 98*:385, 1968.

7. Gould WM, McKeenin DR, Bright R: *Mycobacterium marinum (balnei)* infection. *Arch Derm 97*:189, 1968.

8. Philpott JA, Jr, Woodburne AR, Philpott DS, *et al.* Swimming pool granuloma. *Arch Derm 88*:158, 1963.

9. Sommer AF, Williams RM, Mandel AD: *Mycobacterium balnei* infection. *Arch Derm 86*:316, 1962.

10. Walker HH, *et al*: Some characteristics of "swimming pool" disease in Hawaii. *Hawaii Med J 21*:403, 1962.

11. Samitz MH: *Cutaneous Lesions of the Lower Extremities*. Philadelphia, JB Lippincott, 1971, p 62.

12. Loria PR: Minocycline hydrochloride treatment for atypical acid-fast infection. *Arch Derm 112*:517, 1976.

13. Pillsbury, DM, Shelley WB, Kligman AM: *Dermatology*. Philadelphia, WB Saunders Co, 1956, p 505.

14. Sutton RL Jr: *Diseases of the Skin*. St. Louis, The CV Mosby Co, 1956, p 299.

15. Burnett JW: Uncommon bacterial infections of the skin. *Arch Derm 86*:597, 1962.

16. Lamphier TA: Erysipeloid infection of digits. *J Fla Med Assoc 58*:39, 1971.

17. Taplin D, Bassett DCJ: Foot lesions associated with *Pseudomonas cepacia. Lancet 2*:568, 1971.

X

Dermatitis Caused by
Aquatic Equipment

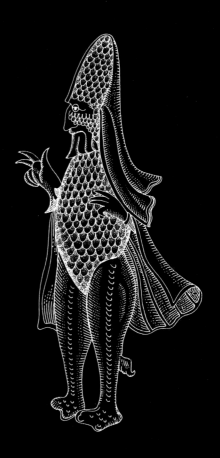

Sea bishop, 16th century Nordic mythology

Dermatitis Caused by Aquatic Equipment

Whirlpool Dermatitis

Recently, physicians in different parts of the country have observed a skin eruption occurring in patients following use of motel whirlpools.[1,2] *Pseudomonas aeruginosa* has been implicated in these dermatoses. It should be noted, however, that *Ps. aeruginosa* is a frequently encountered organism in hotel and motel aquatic facilities; apparently other factors are necessary to produce "whirlpool rash."

Washburn *et al*[1] suggest that inadequate whirlpool disinfection is one of the prime underlying factors. They also cite high whirlpool temperatures that dilate skin pores, high concentrations of pseudomonads, and the presence of chemical irritants as contributory factors.

This group found that 32 of 61 persons who used the swimming pool and whirlpool of a Minnesota motel developed skin lesions. By contrast, no dermatitis or other symptom was reported by 37 motel guests who did not bathe in either of the pools.

In affected patients, the rash appeared 8 to 48 hours after exposure and resolved within seven days without specific treatment. The eruption was described as pruritic, erythematous, maculopapular, and vesiculopustular. While it was most apparent in areas covered by bathing suits, all of the skin areas were affected with the exception of the head and neck. The latter observation strongly implicates the whirlpool as the source of the condition: head and neck areas are likely to be submerged in a swimming pool but not in a whirlpool.

Following the Minnesota outbreak, inspection of the motel's whirlpool disinfecting equipment revealed defective valves and clogged lines. Moreover, the level of free chlorine in the whirlpool was below Minnesota's acceptable level of 0.5 ppm.

Because identification of whirlpool rash is so recent, all data concerning etiology and symptomatology must be considered provisional. Consequently, it is difficult to discuss treatment in any meaningful way. In extremely severe cases, a course of antibiotics should be instituted. Additionally, more stringent monitoring of disinfectant levels may prevent further outbreaks. Physicians encountering patients who appear to have whirlpool-related skin

Pseudomonas aeruginosa has recently been implicated as the cause of so-called whirlpool dermatitis, characterized by a pruritic, papular, pustular eruption.

lesions should report these cases to the proper health authorities so that corrective measures can be taken.

Reactions to Snorkel and Diving Equipment

Another equipment-related dermatologic problem that is observed with increasing frequency is allergic reaction to underwater masks and mouthpieces.

In past years the facial condition known as "mask burn," frequently noted by both physicians and patients, was dismissed as a necessary annoyance of snorkeling and scuba diving. Recently, however, more severe reactions have been described. Although some patients experience only a reddish imprint of the mask on the face, others suffer a severe, painful, and, at times, disabling eruption characterized by vesiculation, weeping, and crusting.

Mouthpieces may result in only minor oral insults without disabling symptoms for lengthy periods. However, patients who become sensitized to the mouthpiece eventually may develop severe intra-oral irritation and inflammation accompanied by vesiculation of the oral mucosa, gingiva, and tongue. Often the initial reaction is a mild burning sensation when the patient drinks hot coffee or tea, fruit juices, or heavily spiced liquids.

Chemical constituents in the equipment may be the causative allergens of these reactions.[3] Rubber masks and mouthpieces con-

Dermatitis and stomatitis due to snorkel or diving equipment may result from allergic hypersensitivity to rubber antioxidants, particularly mercaptobenzothiazol.

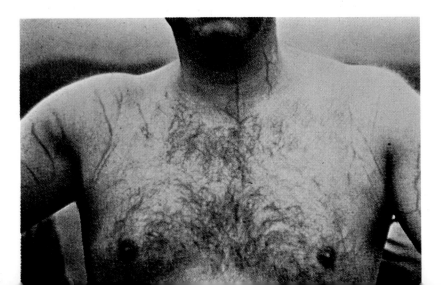

Fig. 10-1. *DIVING SUIT DERMATITIS.* Contact dermatitis of the neck, trunk and extremities due to an allergic reaction to a rubber diving suit.
Courtesy of William Orris, M.D.

tain antioxidants similar to those that are known to cause contact dermatitis in some surgeons following the use of rubber gloves. In particular, mercaptobenzothiazol has caused such instances of rubber dermatitis. Both irritant and allergic reactions to the diving suit may also occur.

Acute facial dermatitis caused by masks should be treated with cold Burow's solution, wet dressings, and systemic corticosteroids.

In serious intra-oral reactions, the patient may obtain symptomatic relief by using a mouth wash consisting of equal parts of an antihistaminic elixir (e.g., diphenhydramine hydrochloride elixir) and milk of magnesia.

For patients who experience severe and frequent reactions, the use of "hypoallergenic" masks and mouthpieces is mandatory. Some manufacturers provide rubber diving equipment which is free of the chemicals to which the diver has proved to have allergic hypersensitivity.

Chapter X— References:

1. Washburn J, Jacobson JA, Marston E, Thorsen B: *Pseudomonas aeruginosa* rash associated with a whirlpool. *JAMA 235*:2205, May 17, 1976.

2. Center for Disease Control: Pool-associated rash illness—North Carolina. *Morbidity Mortality Weekly Rept 24*:349, 1975.

3. Alexander JE: Allergic reactions to mask skirts, regulator mouthpieces, and snorkel mouthpieces. *Pressure 5*:10, Feb 1976.

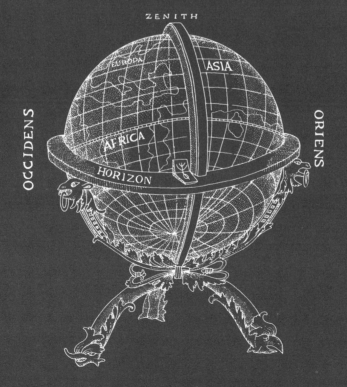

Following is a geographic breakdown—first by location, then by organism—of the water organisms most commonly implicated in dermatologic reactions. Listings are not necessarily all-inclusive, but indicate areas of greatest prevalence as reported in the medical and marine literature. Certain organisms are considered to occur generally in tropical waters, temperate waters, freshwaters or worldwide, etc. These general patterns of distribution are so indicated, in addition to the more specific and most frequently reported areas of habitat.

Geographic Index

Canada, Pacific coast
Schistosome cercariae
Cercaria adamsi
Cercaria columbiensis
Canary Islands
Urchin, sea
Arbacia lixula
Cape Verdi (south to)
Starfish
Echinaster sepositus
Caribbean Sea
Corals
Millepora alcincornis (false, fire, stinging coral)
Fish
Scorpion
Ceylon, coast
Fish
Toadfish
Batrachoides grunniens
China
Cuttlefish
Sepia esculenta (Oriental)
Urchin, sea
Diadoma savignyi (needle-spined urchin)
Cold waters
Norway haddock
Spiny dogfish
Stingray
Weeverfish
Coronado Islands (Mexico)
Schistosome cercariae
Cercaria litterinalinae
Creeks
Leeches
Cuba
Schistosome cercariae
Deeper waters
Sponges
"Poison bun"
Dogger Bank
Sea moss
Sea-chervil
East Africa
Anemone, sea
Rosy anemone
Urchin, sea
Diadema savignyi (needle-spined urchin)
East Africa to Australia
Cone shells
Conus striatus (striated cone)
East Africa to Polynesia
Cone shells

Conus geographus (geographer cone)
Urchin, sea
Heterocentrotus mammillatus
Eastern America, tropical
Worms
Bristle
Hermodice carunculata
England
Starfish
Echinaster sepositus
Estuarial shore lines, temperate (arm of sea, mouth of river, shallow waters)
Louse, sea
Estuarial shore lines, tropical (arm of sea, mouth of river, shallow waters)
Louse, sea
Europe
Cuttlefish
Sepia officinalis (European)
Europe, coast (south)
Fish
Weeverfish
Trachinus vipera (lesser weeverfish)
Florida
Fish
Soapfish
Schistosome cercariae
Florida, coast
Cone shells
Chinese alphabet cone
Conus regius Chemitz
Conus spurius Auct
Queen cone
Florida, east coast
Worms
Bristle
Hermodice carunculata
Florida, St. Petersburg
Sea butterfly
Creseis acicula
Florida Keys
Fish
Scorpion
Sponges
Fire
Worms
Bristle
Hermodice carunculata
France, Atlantic coast
Anemone, sea
Rosy anemone
Freshwaters
Algae

Green
Bacteria
Mycobacterium marinum
Fish
Catfish
Jellyfish
Craspedacusta
Worms
Flatworms
Schistosome cercariae
Gulf of Aden, eastward and through the Atlantic to Red Sea
Corals
Millepora dichotoma (false, stinging)
Gulf of California
Octopus
Octopus fitchi
Worms
Bristle
Chloeia viridis
Gulf of Mexico
Fish
Scorpion
Gulf of Mexico, eastern
Worms
Bristle
Hermodice carunculata
Gulf of Suez
Urchin, sea
Asthenosoma varium (leather urchin)
Hawaii
Algae
Blue-green
Bluebottle
Hawaii, Hilo Bay (Hilo Harbor)
Hydroid, marine
Syncoryne mirabilis
Hawaii to Arabian Sea
Urchin, sea
Phormosoma bursarium
Iceland
Anemone, sea
Rosy anemone
India
Fish
Toadfish
Batrachoides grunniens
Indian Ocean
By-the-wind sailor
Corals
Millepora complanata (false, fire, stinging)

Glaucus atlanticus
Glaucus glaucilla
Octopus
  Octopus maculosus (spotted and
  Hapalochlaena maculosa)
Portuguese man-of-war
Urchin, sea
  Asthenosoma varium (leather
  urchin)
Indian Ocean to Polynesia
Cone shells
  Conus aulicus (court cone)
  Conus marmoreus (marbled cone)
Indo-Pacific
Anemone, sea
  Actinodendron plumosum
Cone shells
  Conus geographus (geographer
  cone)
  Conus striatus (striated cone)
Fish
  Soapfish
Octopus
  Octopus maculosus (spotted and
  Hapalochlaena maculosa)
Portuguese man-of-war
Starfish
  Acanthaster planci
Urchin, sea
  Diadema savignyi (needle-spined
  urchin)
  Heterocentrotus mammillatus
  Phormosoma bursarium
Indonesia
Urchin, sea
  Asthenosoma varium (leather
  urchin)
Japan
Abalone
  Haliotis discus
  Haliotis sieboldi
Cucumber, sea
  Afrocucumus africana
  Polycheira rufescens
  Stichopus japonicus
Cuttlefish
  Sepia esculenta (Oriental)
Octopus
  Octopus defleini
  Octopus maculosus (spotted and
  Hapalochlaena maculosa)
Starfish
  Aphelasterias japonica
  Asterina pectinifera
Urchin, sea

Diadema savignyi (needle-spined
urchin)
Japan, south to Moluccan Sea
Urchin, sea
  Asthenosoma ijimai
Lakes
Algae
  Blue-green
Leeches
Madeira
Urchin, sea
  Arbacia lixula
Malay Archipelago
Cone shells
  Conus gloria-maris (glory of
  the sea)
Fish
  Toadfish
    Batrachoides grunniens
Worms
  Bristle
    Chloeia flava
  Schistosome cercariae
    Cercaria malaya I
    Schistosoma spindule
    ("sawah itch")
Marine waters
Algae
  Blue-green
  Green
Bacteria
  Mycobacterium marinum
Jellyfish
  Chironex fleckeri (sea wasp)
  Chrysaora (sea nettle)
  Cyanea (sea nettle)
Leeches
Portuguese man-of-war
Sea butterfly
Worms
  Bristle
  Flatworms
    Schistosome cercariae
Marine waters, deep
Calycophora
**Mediterranean, northward and through
France to British Isles**
Fish
  Weeverfish
    Trachinus draco
Mediterranean Sea
Anemone, sea
  Rosy anemone
  Sagartia
Fish
  Weeverfish

Trachinus radiatus
Trachinus vipera (lesser
weeverfish)
Octopus
Eledone moschata
Portuguese man-of-war
Starfish
  Echinaster sepositus
Urchin, sea
  Arbacia lixula
Mekong River (Laos)
Fish
  Stingray (freshwater ray)
Mexico
Fish
  Catfish
Mexico, south to Panama
Worms
  Bristle
    Chloeia viridis
Miami area
Sponges
  Fire
Micronesia
Cucumber, sea
  Actinopyga lubrica
Moluccan Sea, north to Japan
Urchin, sea
  Asthenosoma ijimai
Natal Coast
Urchin, sea
  Phormosoma bursarium
New Guinea
Fish
  Toadfish
    Halophryne diemensis
New Zealand
Bluebottle
Schistosome cercariae
  Cercaria longicuada
North Africa
Fish
  Weeverfish
    Trachinus draco
North America
Fish
  Catfish
North Atlantic
By-the-wind sailor
Feather hydroid
Glaucus atlanticus
Glaucus glaucilla
Portuguese man-of-war
North Pacific
By-the-wind sailor

Feather hydroid
Glaucus atlanticus
Glaucus glaucilla
Portuguese man-of-war
North Sea
Fish
Weeverfish
Trachinus vipera (lesser
weeverfish)
**North Sea between Scotland and
Denmark (Dogger Bank)**
Sea moss
Sea-chervil
Norway
Fish
Weeverfish
Trachinus draco
Pacific Ocean, *see also* North Pacific
By-the-wind sailor
Fish
Stingray
Glaucus atlanticus
Glaucus glaucilla
Portuguese man-of-war
Pacific, tropical, *see* Tropical Pacific
Palau
Cucumber, sea
Holothuria axiologa
Panama to Brazil
Fish
Toadfish
Marcgravichthys cryptocentrus
Panama, north to Mexico
Worms
Bristle
Chloeia viridis
Philippines
Chiropsalmus quadrigatus
Cone shells
Conus gloria-maris (glory of
the sea)
Plate River
Fish
Stingray
Polynesia
Starfish
Acanthaster planci
Urchin, sea
Diadema savignyi (needle-spined
urchin)
Polynesia to East Africa
Urchin, sea
Heterocentrotus mammillatus
Cone shells
Conus geographus (geographer
cone)

Polynesia to Indian Ocean
Cone shells
Conus aulicus (court cone)
Conus marmoreus (marbled cone)
Polynesia to Red Sea
Cone shells
Conus textile (textile cone)
Conus tulipa (tulip cone)
Starfish
Acanthaster planci
**Polynesia, westward and through
South Africa to Red Sea**
Cone shells
Conus omaria (pearled cone)
Ponds
Leeches
Pools
Bacteria
Mycobacterium marinum
Puerto Rico
Fish
Soapfish
Red Sea
Anemone, sea
Triactis producta klunzinger
Corals
Millepora complanata (false, fire,
stinging)
Fish
Toadfish
Barchatus cirrhosus
Octopus
Eledone moschata
Starfish
Acanthaster planci
**Red Sea, eastward and through
South Africa to Polynesia**
Cone shells
Conus omaria (pearled cone)
Red Sea to Polynesia
Cone shells
Conus textile (textile cone)
Conus tulipa (tulip cone)
Starfish
Acanthaster planci
**Red Sea, westward and through
Atlantic to Gulf of Aden**
Corals
Millepora dichotoma (false,
stinging)
Running waters
Algae
Blue-green
Ryukyu Islands
Cucumber, sea

Holothuria bivitlata
Saltwater, *see* Marine waters
Seawaters, *see* Marine waters
Sewage treatment systems
Algae
Green
Soil
Bacteria
Mycobacterium marinum
Subtropical waters
By-the-wind sailor
Feather hydroid
Glaucus atlanticus
Glaucus glaucilla
Portuguese man-of-war
Swampy
Bacteria
Pseudomonas cepacia
Tampa Bay
Fish
Stingray
Temperate estuarial shore lines,
see Estuarial shore lines, temperate
Temperate waters
By-the-wind sailor
Glaucus atlanticus
Glaucus glaucilla
Portuguese man-of-war
Temperate zones
Worms
Flatworms
Schistosome cercariae
Tropical estuarial shore lines,
see Estuarial shore lines, tropical
Tropical Pacific
Cone shells
Conus obscurus
Corals
Millepora complanata (false, fire,
stinging)
Tropical rain forest
Leeches
Tropical waters
By-the-wind sailor
Feather hydroid
Glaucus atlanticus
Glaucus glaucilla
Portuguese man-of-war
Worms
Bristle
Euythoe complanata
Tropical zones
Worms
Flatworms
Schistosome cercariae

Synaceja, *see* Fish, Scorpion
Syncoryne mirabilis, *see* Hydroid, marine
Tedania ignis, *see* Sponges, fire
Toadfish, *see* Fish
Triactis producta klunzinger, *see* Anemone, sea
Uncinaria stenocephala, *see* Hookworms
Urchin, sea
    Warm waters
  Araeosoma thetidis (Tam O'Shanter urchin)
    Australia, east coast
  Arbacia lixula
    Africa, west coast
    Azores
    Brazil
    Canary Islands
    Madeira
    Mediterranean Sea
  Asthenosoma ijimai
    Japan, south to Meluccan Sea
  Asthenosoma varium (leather urchin)
    Gulf of Suez
    Indian Ocean
    Indonesia
  Diadema savignyi (needle-spined urchin)
    Africa, east
    Bonin Islands
    China
    Indo-Pacific
    Japan
    Polynesia
  Green
    Caribbean Sea
    Florida
    Florida Keys
    Gulf of Mexico
  Heterocentrotus mammillatus
    Indo-Pacific
    Polynesia to East Africa
  Phormosoma bursarium
    Indo-Pacific
    Hawaii to Arabian Sea
    Natal Coast
Velella velella, *see* By-the-wind sailor
Weeverfish, *see* Fish
Worms, *see also* Schistosome cercariae
  Bristle
    Chloeia flava
      Malayan coast
    Chloeia viridis
      Gulf of California

      Mexico south to Panama
      West Indies
    Euythoe complanata
      Australia
      Tropical seas (tropical zones)
    Hermodice carunculata
      Eastern America, tropical
      Florida, east coast
      Florida Keys
      Gulf of Mexico
  Flatworms
    Arctic
    Freshwaters
    Marine waters
    Temperate zones
    Tropical zones
    Worldwide

Glossary

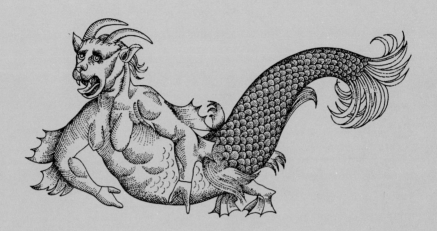

Sea devil, 16th century French mythology

Aboral Opposite to or away from the mouth.

Annelida A phylum of bilateral animals having an epithelium-lined body cavity and including earthworms, bristle worms and leeches. They are distinguished from other worms by the division of their bodies into segments.

Anthozoa A class of marine coelenterates comprising the corals, sea anemones and related forms distinguished by polyps with radial partitions or mesenteries projecting from the body wall into the gastrovascular cavity.

Barbel Diminutive of barb, particularly as applied to barbs of fish. Also the soft-finned freshwater fish *Barbus fluviatilis*.

Bivalve Having a shell composed of two usually movable valves that open and shut. An animal with two valved shells, especially a mollusk of the class Lamellibranchia (as a clam, mussel or oyster).

Calcareous Pertaining to chalk or to its color or texture.

Cephalopoda A class of mollusks containing the squids, cuttlefish and octopus, and characterized by the fact that the foot is drawn out into tentacles surrounding the head.

Cercaria A tadpole-shaped larval trematode worm. It is usually produced in the molluscan host and later freed into water to penetrate a suitable definitive host.

Chitin A white or colorless amorphous horny substance that forms part of the hard outer integument of insects, crustaceans, and some other invertebrates. It occurs also in fungi, being a polysaccharide structurally similar to cellulose.

Coelenterata A phylum of the animal kingdom distinguished by the presence of nematocysts (stinging capsules), a diploblastic body wall in Hydrozoa, and a single internal cavity opening to the exterior only at the oral end. So defined, the phylum comprises the Hydrozoa, jellyfish, corals and sea anemones, but

excludes the Ctenophora (comb-jellies) that lack nematocysts.

Conidae A very large family of gastropod mollusks deriving their name from the cone-shaped shells characterized by a large conical body whorl under a short blunt turret. Many tropical Conidae have a venomous bite.

Coral Any marine coelenterate that produces a calcareous skeleton.

Coral head A rounded, often knobby protuberance of coralline material on the submerged portion of a coral reef, or in close proximity to it.

Coral reef Marine structure, made up chiefly of fragments of corals, coral sands, algae and other organic deposits, and the solid limestone resulting from their consolidation.

Crustacea A large class of the phylum Arthropoda including the crabs, lobsters, shrimps, beach hoppers, sow bugs, barnacles, water fleas and allied forms. They may be distinguished from other arthropod classes by the possession of two pairs of preoral antennae. Most possess at least three pairs of postoral appendages functioning as jaws, and almost all are aquatic.

Cubomedusae An order of jellyfish distinguished by a generally cubic form.

Diatom Common name of Bacillariophyceae, a class of tiny one-celled or aggregate planktonic algae having silicified skeletons that form the material diatomite.

Echinodermata That phylum of the animal kingdom which contains the sea urchins, sea stars, sea cucumbers, and sea lillies. They are distinguished by a radial symmetry of five, and a calcareous skeleton usually consisting of external spine-bearing plates.

Elasmobranch Pertaining to a class of fishes having lamellate gills and including sharks and rays. The class is also distinguished by a cartilaginous skeleton, which in larger forms sometimes becomes calcified, but never ossified.

Gastropoda That class of mollusks which comprises the snails, slugs and whelks. They are distinguished by their well-developed head, and generally by an elongate conical shell coiled in a spiral.

Hirudinea A class of annelid worms commonly called leeches. They are distinguished by the absence of bristles and the presence of suckers.

Holothurioidea A class of Echinodermata commonly called sea cucumbers. They are distinguished by their elongate shape and reduction of the skeleton to spicules or plates embedded in the leathery body wall.

Hydrozoan Pertaining to a class of coelenterates comprising simple and compound polyps, and jellyfishes lacking gastric tentacles.

Intertidal Of, relating to, or being a part of the littoral zone that is above low-tide mark.

Isopoda An order of small crustaceans, commonly known as sea lice, that live as parasites on invertebrates and fish. They are distinguished by the absence of a carapace, and by a body usually divided into seven free thoracic segments, each bearing a pair of similar legs.

Liverwort A marine plant related to and resembling the mosses, but differing in reproduction and development.

Mollusca A phylum of bilateral invertebrates comprising the clams, oysters, snails, whelks, squids and octopuses. They are characterized by a soft unsegmented body; many secrete a calcareous shell.

Nectocalyx A free-swimming "bell" of a siphonophore (*see* Siphonophora).

Nectophore *See* nectocalyx.

Nematocyst One of the minute stinging organs of certain jellyfish and related coelenterates.

Nettle cell *See* Nematocyst.

Nudibranchiata A suborder of gastropods commonly called sea-slugs. The name derives from the dorsal respiratory extension of the mantle, often brilliantly colored.

Oscula A characteristic feature of the sponge bearing one or more conspicuous rounded openings or vents.

Pedicellaria One of numerous, minute, usually two or three "fingered" pincerlike organs, found on the surface of many echinoderms.

Pelecypoda The "shellfish" class of mollusks distinguished by their bivalved shells and including clams, oysters and mussels.

Porifera The phylum of the animal kingdom which contains the sponges. In general they consist of aggregates of cells that line canals and chambers, and are usually supported by a skeleton of fibers or spicules.

Proboscides The anterior muscular protrusible part of the alimentary canal of many annelids.

Pteropoda A separate class of small hermaphroditic gastropod mollusks, including the sea butterfly, having the anterior lobes of the foot expanded into winglike organs with which they swim at or near the surface of the sea. They usually lack gills, and frequently lack a shell.

Radula A ribbon-like band bearing transverse rows of teeth found about the mouth in many mollusks.

Ray Any of numerous elasmobranch fishes having a dorsoventrally flattened body, with mouth and gill clefts on the lower surface and eyes on the upper surface, usually enormously developed pectoral fins arrayed continuously along the margin of the head and body, and a typically slender whip-like caudal process often equipped with venomous spines. Rays are adapted for life on the sea bottom, and feed chiefly on mollusks which they crush with blunt, flattened teeth.

Schistosoma A genus of the family Schistosomatidae comprising digenetic, elongated trematode worms that can penetrate and parasitize the blood vessels of man and other mammals.

Scombroid A subfamily of food fishes distinguished by a deeply forked tail and spiny fins, and comprising the tuna, mackerel, bonito, and swordfish.

Scorpaenidae A large family of carnivorous, usually bottom-dwelling, marine spiny-finned fishes comprising the lionfish, zebrafish, bullrout, waspfish and other scorpion fishes. They most typically possess one or more pairs of spiniferous ridges on the head and a dorsal fin supported by strong spines which in some forms have poison glands and inflict severe wounds.

Sea butterfly *See* Pteropoda.

Sea cucumber A holothurian, esp. any holothurian whose contracted body suggests a cucumber in form.

Sea louse *See* Isopoda.

Sea urchin An echinoderm of somewhat flattened globular form, having a thin brittle shell or covering of calcareous plates, and distinguished from the disk-shaped sand dollars or cake urchins and the heart urchins by an "armor" of well developed and often very sharp, movable spines.

Scyphozoa A class of coelenterate comprising jellyfishes that have endodermal gastric tentacles, endodermal gonads which discharge their products into the digestive cavity, and which can regenerate asexually.

Sea anemone Any non-skeletogenous coelenterate having radially partitioned polyps.

Siphonophora An order of Hydrozoa consisting of various free-swimming transparent and often showily colored forms usually regarded as compound animals. They are composed of zooids modified to perform specialized functions for the colony (as feeding, defense,

locomotion), and may have two or more zooids in the form of a bell which by their contractions cause the colony to swim.

Spongin A scleroprotein which is the chief constituent of the flexible skeletal fibers of commercial sponges and certain other sponges.

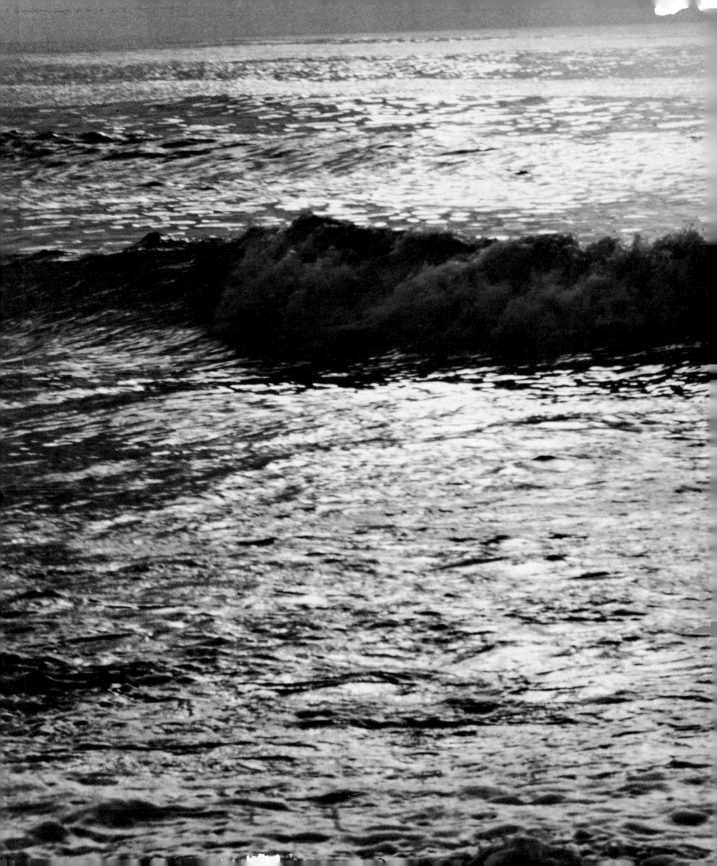